Chapter One

August 4, 1778

The forest extended across the ancient mountains and was only broken by the Susquehanna River, which weaves its way through them. For eons, the thriving trees that covered the land's timeless face protected the lives of those living beneath them. Eons of time that extended into the ages. Ages that witnessed all the lives pass through them with patience born from the earth.

> None of the living things in the dark forests seemed so among them.

resilient as people. They forged trails through the forest tapestry, with their charming hamlets or villages covering the riverbanks occasionally, slightly scaring the land and the ages.

> Others came into this forest and the ancient Native American order.

From lands far away across the oceans. They blew like a new wind. The Native peoples feared it would forever alter the nature of the land. The newcomers were able to turn their hearts in a completely different direction. Their hearts were different. Their minds thought differently. Their passions drove them to a

Different way. Through their eyes, or white eyes as ancient peoples called it, a new light shone and changed everything.

> Native peoples attempted to resist the wind blowing.

These newcomers were able to see the white eyes of the Native people, but they also had a fever that few have ever seen. The British and Native

Americans gave them battle. It was a terrible battle that would have driven an inferior people with lesser passions away forever. The Battle of Wyoming, July 3, 1778.

These newcomers, these white-eyed Wyoming settlers, are not so fortunate.

They called themselves. Let the passions that fueled them fuel their lives. They returned to the place of the battle, the Wyoming Valley, because these passions drove them. The land they now call their blessed land, which was taken by the Native people and Tories only a few months before, is still alive with the passions of the terrible Battle of Wyoming.

This is the clash of passions that occurred between Wyoming settlers, and Indians.

The Battle of Wyoming had not brought an end to the Tories, their allies. They were conservative Americans who did no rebel against their God-given sovereign. It would not end, however, as it did in the larger Revolutionary War. The heart of the last Wyoming man was cut off and his blood sank into the ground he loved.

Many of them tried to oppose the Six Nations and their leaders.

Allies lay in the Wyoming fields* until this day, and they are still there. As they walked along the trail back towards Wyoming, this thought haunted all the settler. But they continued to walk. Their ragged but determined column of men held a variety of firelocks with their white-knuckled fists. Their headgear was as diverse as their clothing.

There was no sound except for the tired shuffle of the feet.

It should not betray their presence, which might be their foe, who might just be behind any bush or tree that is poised to strike.

That meant that every shadow was given the attention it deserved by those who were on the other side.

For the reminders of that terrible battle a month ago, the flanks of the settlers' marching men were tightly packed in single file along the narrow trail.

Wyoming was, at the American Revolution, the area that ran along the Susquehanna River, from Tioga Point (present Athens Pa.) to Nescopeck Pa.

They were able to see something new, something that they could not erase. Every noise they heard from the shadows provoked a new reaction, a new fear. However, this was quickly quelled when an animal flew in the direction of the sound.

Although they were tempted by the idea of using their meager and stale food to kill the deer, turkey, squirrels and other wildlife, they saw along the trailside that not one shot was heard from them. Their veins were tingling with hunger, but they knew better. Their colonel did not need to remind them a hundred times about the importance of getting to the valley as quietly as possible. Their colonel had plans to announce their arrival to the rest of the world once they had reclaimed their home. Attention Tories! Beware of the Six Nations! Wyoming is back! The threat of ambush was too constant to ignore. They all learned this lesson from Wyoming's bloody battlefield of death.

The trail's familiar sights evoked images of happier and more fulfilling times.

More hopeful times, but now clouded with the terrible retreat from the battle that ended it all. Some of these men fought along the trail to the refuge of the settlements on the Delaware River with their children and wives, just weeks ago. Their determination fuelled a burning desire for revenge in their exhausted souls.

They had trod it in defeat. They now trod it in defiance

To reclaim their homes and lives, their land, their dignity, and their dignity. Once they have regained their foothold, no one will force them to leave the ground. No.

True, they felt a hollow and empty feeling of doubt.

They may have a few thoughts from time to others, but they only need to look at their coworkers to get rid of them. Each man sees the sternness in his soul through his eyes. Fear resisted it. It confirmed the determination that was burning within each one of them. John Jenkins saw Obadiah Gore, who was marching alongside him. Luke Swetland, an older man with keen eyes, turned to Isaac Tripp, his friend from high school. Moses Brown looked to Ira Stephens, a veteran of many battles. Nathan Denison did look to Zebulon Butler.

They saw something in their eyes that reaffirmed the cursed spirit

Through all their veins. The spirit of the pioneer, it, was difficult to describe verbally. It could only be felt by others of the same spirit. This spirit fought against reality and allowed certain people to overcome seemingly impossible odds and win. This spirit was so strong in these Americans that it seemed to inspire and enrich them all the way across the continent. Only then did the south seas stop them.

However, not everyone, even some American friends, shares the same spirit. These

Others mocked and jeered the pioneers, calling their spirit foolish folly. These words were spoken even in Connecticut by some. They pulsated through the bodies of many, from their tired feet to their aching head. You are now dead! You are a fool! Recover your losses and go home! Don't leave the forest to the savages They have already beaten you! He is a fool for his folly!

These words are spoken in warm hearts in distant hamlets.

These men felt hollow as they walked along the coast. Some spoke, while others acted. People who spoke only rarely understood those who did not speak, those who acted on the words they spoke.

Wyoming Valley is a beautiful, pristine area that seems to be everywhere.

It must be reclaimed, graced by God's hand. It must be saved. It was too bloody and too precious to be ignored. Their sweat and blood stained the land. Their blood was their lifeblood. It was unquestionably theirs. The promise of Wyoming was far more important than the horrors and consequences of war. Their safe and warm homes also made it a risky war. It is better to fight it here by men of such spirit than by those whose lives are too comfortable to make the sacrifices that war requires.

Both their land and lives were forever intertwined.

Their enemies, the British Crown and the Six Nations, held it in their hands. They must march to recover it and fight again for it if necessary. The talkers and others will not be able to understand. These people, who are also overcome by reason, will never understand it. But the doers like General Washington understood and promised relief. They found faith and trust in this man. They may be ridiculed by the rest of the country, but men made from the same fabric understand. Their understanding is all that they need.

The troops' tired pace suddenly became more lively. Heads perked up,

They rose from their chests. They looked at the burned buildings in front of them with concern. Silently, they filed around the desolated farmstead, spreading out along the sides of the trail. The men spread out among the trees, with their firelocks ready to strike at any unwary foe. To their horror, no Indians were able to haunt the forest in the wake of this cruel act.

Slowly, a single horseman trotted through the charred buildings.

lower lip rising in disgust. His mount's feet ran across the litter of iron pots and bits of once-precious china, torn featherbeds and other tools of an once prosperous and promising past. He brought his mount to a halt beside the carcass and bones of rotten beef, its legs sticking straight up from the ground. He almost fell to his knees from the rancid smell. He noticed the trail of wolf tracks that led from the carcass to dense woods beyond. His jaw tightened and he let out a low grunt.

One lone wolf suddenly began to cry in the still air. It seemed to be answering his question.

It may scoff or vent its anger at being interrupted during its feast.

Alert eyes scanned the area for the sound and grabbed their surroundings.

Rifles in their white-fisted knuckles. The wolf, a warrior for opportunity, would die if it showed up, just like its adversaries. The forest's dark corners did not conceal its presence.

Everybody stood and looked in the direction the eerie howl was directing.

It was a question of whether it could be a bad sign or not. A few whispered a prayer. The horseman grunted disapproval and reached for the pistol, which was still in his belt.

The lone howl became a chorus of howls.

Instigated and facilitated by the forest Gods' painted demons. The horseman raised his gun in the air and fired. His mount was anxiously following his lead until his firm hand tightened its reins. With the retreating wolves, the howls faded slowly. He cleverly reined his horse around, facing the wide-eyed men in front of him.

He looked around, trying to gauge each man's continence using their

eyes. He nodded and tucked his pistol back into his belt. He finally spoke, breaking the awkward silence. "Men," said he, adding, "Look around you!" Not to forget, Bullock's Farm is nine miles from the actual valley. Take a look at the destruction! "I hope you find the same strength in your resolve that I have!

He was answered by a few, but not one of them spoke.

He placed his hand on the pommel of the saddle and pushed it down.

He straightened his long frame by placing it in the saddle. He sat tall and straight in the saddle, looking at the charred buildings. He was silently grateful that no human skeletons were among the destruction. He looked around for his home in the valley and turned to go.

He shouted, "Lieutenant Jenkins!" "Mr. Hollenback! To the front at once!"

Two men jumped out of the ranks of the soldiers who were milling,

They are followed by dozens of people.

"Yes sir Colonel Butler," both men replied at once, snapping to

Pay attention to him.

"Each of the you are to gather ten men of your choosing to

reconnoiter the Valley, you Jenkins, from north, and you Hollenback from south." He stopped, looking over his shoulder at the remains of the farmstead. He said, "If you come across any devils, do what you can." "The rest will make their way to the river common, and we'll meet you there. The day is getting longer, so be diligent in your work.

Momentarily, both men raised their right hand to the brims.

They hung up their hats and turned to face the eager faces, begging to be included in their ranks. They quickly filled their ranks with nods and pointed fingers. They quickly gathered their men and checked their weapons and accoutrements. They rushed off to the farmstead in a split second, one in each direction and the other in the opposing direction. Their dispirited eyes were focused on their departure.

Butler advised them to "Don't worry." "There will be sport."

We all must continue to march until this issue is resolved! Now, let's get back on the road! This is only the first step. Be careful with each step. Our enemies could lurk around us. The sun hasn't set yet on their empire. Be aware that the curse of tomahawks prevails! We may win and strike their hearts with a fatal blow. This may prove to be the only way to end it all. For our wives, children, homes, dignity, and country, we must move on!

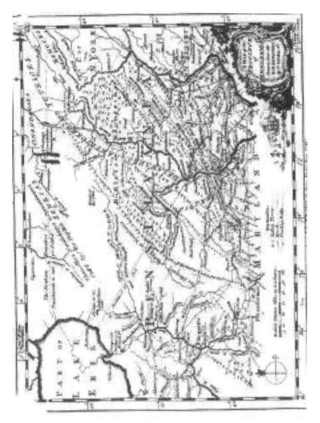

Chapter Two

Matthias Hollenback kept his eyes fixed on the summit of the mountain in front of him and he walked with all his might towards the summit. He knew Colonel Butler and the other men would be following him so he wanted to get their van cleared as quickly as possible. His keen eyes searched all around him.

His mind was filled with worry for the men who followed him, as he knew them all and trusted their keen eyes.

They trotted together without a word being spoken between them. Each man

He was a keen observer of the hunt and shared his enthusiasm for it with his companion. They were the first patriots ever to walk on Wyoming soil. They were terrified of that honor.

They were all enemies, no matter how many they were.

Each followed Hollenback's lead silently, but a Pennamite bystander

Birth, a Yankee heart beat within his chest. His trade skills and ambition made him a successful businessman and he was a great friend to his fellow traders. His shirt was stained by blood from an injury sustained in battle. This wound was exacerbated by his courageous trek to regain Wyoming.

He finally reached the summit of the mountain and stopped. All was gathered

He looked down at the green valley below from his circle of friends. The Susquehanna looked radiant in the sunlight, likening it as a silver thread weaving through the green tapestry God's earth. From the Nanticoke Falls rapids, crests of water rose against its silvery face. The gentle breezes blew the mountain in front of them and an eagle flew along them. They were beautiful, but their eyes didn't see the beauty. It was those who were trampling it.

Hollenback took his hat and wiped his forehead. "None

"As I see, they are all about," he stated, raising his rifle's pan to his front to check for powder. He added, gesturing down the mountainside to a small clearing at the foot. "We'll go down to the clearing, then we'll turn north. If ye see rats, they can have it!"

> Each man spreads out in a straight line and each man is a few arms lengths away from the other.

They both descended into the valley. They moved slowly, as usual, and all jumped when the sound of a turkey taking its wings sounded. In its madness, a few curses were uttered. Hollenback forced a hard swallow to his dry throat and motioned them towards a large boulder sticking out of the mountainside. The rocks provided a little respite from the forest, and gave them a good vantage point to view their goal. He waved his men to the river's edge, hoping that their dirty and worn-out clothes would conceal them from the curious eyes.

> He said, painfully conscious of the late hour: "Cast your eyes around."

The sun was already reaching the summit of the mountain behind them. His fear was heightened by the deep breaths and pantless men. He was wrong. The mountain was steeper than he expected. However, he had to cover more ground.

> He curses himself for forgetting to say a curse under his breath

In his haste to find spyglass, he glanced at the green sea that covered the mountains. He thought that the glass would have been very useful. He noticed a particularly fast series of pants and turned his attention to the older man behind them. He was well over ten years older than the rest of the group and now showed it. He leaned against the tree, pure and simple exhaustion.

"Look smart, my dear man," Hollenback said.

The man bowed his heads. "Spirit's willing," said he, panting. "But it plays hell on your body sometimes." He looked around to find someone who shared his humor, but only stern eyes stared at him.

Hollenback stated, "We must stand up to our work Giles.".
Giles Slocum was still panting and tried to suppress an inappropriate laugh. He rubbed his palm on a spot on the trunk of the tree next to him, but it was not enough. He said, "Damn them porcupines." "They'll decimate many a good tree if they have to." This one is gnawing at me. They will gnaw and chew for months, and then you'll know that the tree isn't going to be leafing any more. It's true, I swear it.

Hollenback raised an eyebrow at the man. Some men might say

Anything in stressful moments. Their laughter seemed to calm their nerves. In the heat of battle at Wyoming, he recalled hearing men shouting and firing. He didn't care if they fired more, it was irrelevant to him. He didn't take any such into consideration, but knowing the horrors Slocum had suffered on the battlefield, he allowed it to pass.

Slocum did not pay any attention to their indifference. It was a great time being out there

On a man's heart. A memory can bring light to a moment. He continued, "Damned Porcupines," and let a smile grow on the surface. He laughed inappropriately, but he will never forget Grandpa Tripp's night in the privy. "Got quilled he did. No lie, some of us might recall if we have the time. Grandpa Tripp shouted loud enough to wake Queen Ester up at Tioga Point. I yelled like a stuck porcupine! You know what, damm porcupines hate salt from the drippings around the hole. However, Grandpa howled even more when Hooker Smith pulled the quills out of his foot. They weren't in his foot either!"

He was stern, but his smiles were a lightening bolt. Humor worked,

The serious mood was lit. There were a few laughs in the air.

Hollenback answered, with a serious tone, "Yes", and he looked up at the smiles of the pioneers. "Let's not get sidetracked! "Not by a quill but an Indian lance!"

Slocum nodded with the others and choked down his desire.

To laugh again. He lifted his rifle, and after catching his exhaling breaths, he moved off the tree, giving the tree's bare spot one more rub. Under his breath, he murmured to himself "Damn those porcupines.".

Hollenback told him, "Like I've stated, a quill is nothing compared to the spear.".

Slocum did not say anything more and was replaced by others scanning

the river bottom below.

Hollenback seemed keener in his eyes. He stared at the ground with intense interest.

He did not glance at the ground, but carefully surveyed each yard. He didn't miss a shadow or a bush. All his senses had to be sharp because of the potential danger of ambush. He cursed himself for having forgotten his spyglass. It was so bizarre! He quickly retorted. It's okay. They all carry full cartridge boxes, full powder horns and lots of lead. He reassured himself that he, and any of his men would fall to the savage today. It's now the Indians who will fall.

The valley below was left empty, save for a few.

He motioned his men forward once more, whether they were deer, wolves, or elk. He said, "We don't see anything, but we have our firelocks ready, who knows what lurks in the shadows?" Another turkey snuck up to their front and startedled the rifles that followed it. They lowered their heads, staring at the captain with an anxious gaze.

He said, "It's okay." "I'm glad that you are all so eager to drop anything."

Which wears a feather?" He noticed the shadows getting deeper and the sun sinking behind the mountain more. He added, "Let's make for the river with all due haste. That is where we will find some sport if any." He looked back at the older men and saw that the most eager eyes were the younger ones. We will follow if you are young and agile.

The younger men were satisfied with that. They poured down

The setting sun made the mountainside swell with a rush. Twigs snapped and some stumbled, but no one stopped for a second. Solomon Bennett, a young man, was the one who has gotten further ahead. He lost himself in the race's momentum and burst into a clearing at bottom of mountain, his comrades behind him. There were thorns in both his legs and arms that he wanted to pay attention to. He lowered his rifle to tend them. A slight movement in his corner caused him to instinctively lift it again. His jaw dropped at the sight three tall forest warriors. He quickly raised his rifle from his shoulder. He was barely breathing and his nervous fingers pulled the trigger of his rifle towards the stunned faces of the warriors.

The white apparition bearing down upon them was stared at by the warriors.

As if out of nowhere, in stunned disbelief. What magic made the white demon appear from thin air? Astounded, they stood. Two of them frozen in the motion of loading a fresh killed deer into a canoe, while the third held a bundle of cloth in his hands and looked down at three rifles at their feet.

As you reach down, you see a sudden puff of smoke that is both blue and white.

His face was smashed into the ground, and he fell backwards against his stunned companions. His upper chest exploded, soaking the canoe in red. Twisting, he rolled through pure agony through his friends' hands and into the swirling Susquehanna with the canoe next to him.

Two stunned Indians muttered a confused yell, and then they jumped up in dismay.

Mixed with angry curses echoing down to the mountain. The mountainside was stricken by a mad rush. The mad rush of Yankees. Copperheads curse! Copperheads! The once peaceful forest was ravaged by the Copperheads! The mountain was sprayed with Yankee fury.

"I got them!" Bennett shouted, "I got 'em!"

He stood wide-eyed, furiously trying load his gun. "Come quick! Come quick!"

More roars answered him.
The eyes of the braves darted around to see everything, from their rifles to the canoe.

And to their flailing comrades in the swirling waters. The bigger of the two cried and madly gestured towards the canoe, breaking his companion's gaze on the rifles. He reached out and grabbed the canoe with one of his large hands, while encouraging the other to follow his lead using his tongue. The other brave pulled his tomahawk out of his belt and flung it at the white, wide-eyed demon in frustration.

The weapon flew harmlessly, and the demon quickly dodged.

He pushed the brush behind him. The white demon ran madly and rammed it home with his rifle.

They were brave, only a matter of seconds apart.

Another assault was made, as the paddler wildly pushed the canoe along the river, throwing the deer into the turbulent waters. The brave man in the rear threw his paddle from one end of the canoe onto the other, paddling for his life. His bigger partner struggled with the wounded man's hand and tried to help him paddle against the water. He finally managed to lift the injured man out of the water and he poured him into the canoe. Both hands grabbed the paddle quickly.

The canoe was surrounded by a hail of lead. Near misses of splinters striking the rail caused them to fly. It was surrounded by little gouts. The braves raised their paddles and prayed to reach the shore before the shots of mad demons buzzing through the air stung.

Hollenback ran down the mountain in an anxious race to get his order.

Advance pell-mell may not be a disaster. You fool! He thought to himself, he was going against his better judgement and all. He listened to the gunshots below and tried to figure out how many men were being enthralled by the sound. He finally reached the foot of the mountain and burst into the clearing, relieved at the sight in front of him.

All men standing in any position were fired against

To help them aim, they could either kneel or lie flat on the ground. Each quickly rammed a ball home and fired again. Smoke filled the clearing.

Hollenback jumped to the front of men, looking through the windows.

smoke. Two brave men dragged another man up the far shore, trying to escape the lead's deadly hail. He instinctively raised the rifle and fired. He watched as the warriors disappeared into the forest, peering through the smoke. He gasped in frustration knowing that they would not be found.

He yelled, "That's it boys!" "They're gone once they gain the

We will never find sugar bush they are not there!"

One of them shouted "To hell with it!" and fired blindly into the air.

Trees on the other shore.

Hollenback told him, "That's enough!" Hollenback scolded him.

Powder and lead in your pouch to fight the Six Nations in their entirety

"No, but I'll damn certain put a hurting on those red-skinned devils.

sees!" the man countered.

"You can't play safe with your life, but you should not be playing without consequences."

Hollenback said, looking deathly at Hollenback, and leaving no doubt about his sincerity.

The man dropped his rifle and spit in frustration on the ground. He said, "Rifle's about fowled anyway." "Damn Continental powder anyways!" All the powder Colonel Stroud had kept for Fort Penn was used by him anyway! He didn't want any powder wasted on the Yankees who braved the forest to return their land. Stroud doesn't care how! He's not his land! Damn Pennamite rascal!"

"They must have come out for their canoe as we were starting down."

"From the rocks," a man reported lifting up some branches from the shore. "Had they hidden their game under them and returned to fetch it. They are clever devils. You never know when or where they will appear.

Hollenback nodded. He hoped that the man would give an accurate appraisal of their enemy.

He struck a chord with his men because every word rang true. Bennett was able to smile and lighten the mood. You did well! You still got your hair! Are you the one who hit it?

Bennett smiled with beaming eyes and said "Yes sir." Bennett nodded and nodded.

He quickly acknowledged the praises of those around him.

One of the Indians' rifles that had been abandoned by the Indians was saved by another man.

hands. He said, "These aren't trade rifles." They're fine rifles if they are properly made and taken care of.

They gathered together, thinking but not speaking, and they all thought about each other.

feared. It is not difficult to believe that the weapons were obtained from Wyoming's battlefield.

Hollenback asked, "Do you all recognize them?".
Shaking heads answered him.
"Looks like your prize will float away boy," said a grinning looking

Buckskin-clad man said it, pointing his rifle barrel at the river. The canoe moved along the shore. It was being pushed by the current, which threatened to sweep it away at any moment.

Bennett looked at the exquisitely made Birch Bark Canoe.

groaning. He imagined the treasure inside it and his imagination ran wild. In anticipation, he looked up to Hollenback.

"Damn!" Hollenback said. Hollenback said, "Damn!"

It's up to you. It's your choice.

Bennett exclaimed, quickly removing his shoes.

shirt. "Can't let it pass."

He led everyone to the shore. He stripped off everything.

He waded into water with his buckskin britches.

One of the men called out to him, reaching for a knife. "Keep this between your teeth for safety."

Bennett grabbed the item eagerly and bit down. He turned and didve.

Swimming with all his might against strong currents, he plunged into the water.

Hollenback directed the rest of the order: "Everyone load up and stand ready."

The men. "If there is anything more than a damn chipmunk showing itself over there, blister it!"

All stood with guns raised and watched. Soon, the boy was freed.

He rushed to the canoe's edge and climbed down, hurriedly. It began to move and release its precarious hold at the shoreline, allowing it to drift towards Nanticoke Falls in the swift current.

Bennett quickly grabbed a paddle and sank it in the water. Bennett quickly raised a paddle and sank it into the water.

He was greeted by a crowd of people who were happy to see him return on the other riverbank. He was the winner of the first Wyoming victory and had the trophy to prove it. Although it seemed all was well for a brief moment, each man didn't take much stock in the feelings. This is only the beginning, Colonel Butler stated.

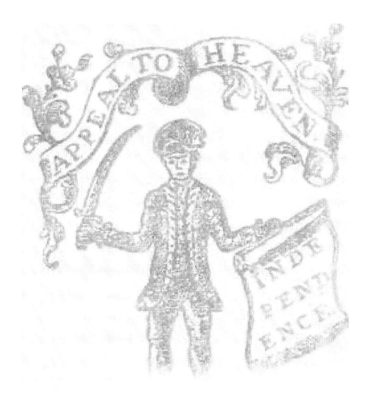

Chapter Three

The men followed the river at Wilkes-Barre and their nervous eyes soon turned to dismay at what they saw. There was nothing but the charred remains from many homes, except for one cabin that they naturally found. The shock of realizing their enemy's strength and terrible resolve made stunned men fall into a daze. Others wandered aimlessly, dragging their rifles behind their backs in limp hands, and staring in shock at the places that once held their heart. They looked at the burned homes that had once sheltered and nurtured many children within their walls. They had lost everything that was once their future. All their hopes and dreams were gone. More than just their homes, the flames had also destroyed them. They had also destroyed people's lives. Their lives. Their families' lives.

Zebulon Butler rode slowly on his horse around the streets ravaged by fire.

His mind was also racing with thoughts. He was surrounded by an enormous elm tree that he was shivering from the memories of many of his friends and family members who had spent many summer days under its shade, sharing their hopes and dreams for a better tomorrow. Tomorrow is always tomorrow. They had already built a sanctuary in the wilderness, and they could do it again. Many of the fields still had grain, which was likely left behind by the enemy for future use. It would soon ripen, and the enemy might return with it. No! Too many people depended on the grain, including the ones who planted it. Many faced poverty and destitution without it.

He suddenly jumped out of his saddle and walked over to the cabin. He lifted his hand and pressed against one of the corners of the cabin's charred timbers. The wood creaked, but it remained firm. He was surrounded by curious, but still sulky men who heard the noise.

He said, "See", to them, while putting his hand on his thigh. "It's charred but its heart is still solid!" Not unlike us! Although it's not much, it's something.

The men looked down as they slowly moved back towards the front.

The cabin. A few others also struck flint to light a fire in the pit. They sat down and blew on tinder, always mindful of the shadows growing and disregarding their prancing colonel.

Butler ignored their indifference and approached Denison, his old friend. He was leaning against a tree, looking at the men trying to light the fire. He had never seen a man so brokenhearted. He said, "Come now

Nathan." "The fields are still full, and the grain, and harvest, don't forget them. It will be a new beginning made from the ashes. We are glad we went into the wilderness to find a way home. It is not up to the Indians and Tories to take it!

It is not possible to leave it up to the Pennamites!"

Denison murmured, "Ashes," as he rubbed his lips against his tongue. "All

is ashes and forsaken."

Butler pulled his horse closer and leaned forward from the saddle.

Observe his eyes closely. Could this be the staunch defender for the valley? What about the men if his spirit was ravaged? He must act before all men are affected by the grief and lose all hope. Dear friend, get a grip on yourself. We are all alone out there. He said it loud enough to his friend.

Through long strands, his blank and empty eyes gazed back at him.

Under a worn and frayed slouch, Denison wore his sweat-soaked locks of hair. Denison mumbled, "But all is lost," and he neglected to brush his hair in front of his eyes. "We barely have enough provisions to get back to Fort Penn. It was all I could do now to get the arms this rabble had, and many of them I don't doubt will shoot straight at me. Stroud was a formidable opponent that I had to fight hand and foot! These men are not fools, but they are brave! Maybe it's all foolishness! What should we do if Indian Butler returns only with a third?

"We'll fight to have that rascal's hair before it is all."

done!" Butler said.

Denison stated, "Bold words", "I have heard them before,"

Lazarus Stewart's lips are no less.

Butler's eyes widen at the mention that the brash captain whom he was is

He had demanded they marche out to meet the enemy in the final battle, while Denison and he cautioned against it. They preferred to wait for reinforcements. He was a brave soldier who had fallen on battle's field; Wyoming settler should not lose that honor. However, to suggest that he had behaved as recklessly cut deeply into his pride.

"I will never speak poorly of any of the dead on the battlefield,"

He said that all had died with honor. "But we can't just die and lay down. It is a shame for their memory as well as ours.

"I arrested him, and would have tried to have him tried if you wouldn't have."

Denison stated, "I intervened when it was your turn." "You, of all people. The irony of it all."

"I wouldn't have marched out the way I did if it wasn't for his influence.

true," Butler said. Butler said, "But I am not to blame." You and no one else. It would have been much more different if I had fought correctly, waited for Franklin and Clingman's men, sent the militia out to draw in the Tory rats, and all that was required of me. That is all! There is nothing we can do about it right now. I, however, honor those brave souls now and forever. "That is all I will ever say about the matter!" He looked up at the dimming sky and sighed.

"Now, my man, it's for us who live to remember those who died and reclaim the things they gave all for, their children, wives and yes, even for us all."

The stirring words did not have any effect. Denison rubbed his forehead.

The trunk of the tree is what he collides with. He asked, "What words are there in the face of such a thing?".

Butler looked at the other men with anxious eyes. He could not bear to lose Denison.

He had lost everything. He clutched his hands tightly to his saddle horn and searched his mind for something that would revive his frail ranks. He fought back against his anger but his frustration turned into anger. His ragged clothes caught his attention. His trousers, shirt and waistcoat were torn apart by thorns and scrub brush. His body started to feel charred, with bruises and aches. He gasped and shook his head as he felt the despair sweep over him. He lowered his head to his chest and let his hat drop to the ground. He looked at the hat, but felt drained of energy to lift it up.

A roar suddenly erupted at the river's edge. Men perked up

They stepped away from the fire and looked at the disturbance in readiness to face the new threat. They quickly formed a line and aimed their firelocks at the riverbank.

A voice yelled, "Hold on there!" Mathias Hollenback, it is!

We are back with a smart prize!

The rifles fell. The party was full of excitement for Hollenback's men

They rushed to the riverbank and rallied their friends, so full of life they didn't seem to notice the faces of the fallen. They rushed up to the fire and plopped several turkeys that they had shot. All of them wore wide eyes and smiled from ear to toe. The jubilant men quickly spread their emotions through the other turkey hunters, exchanging congratulatory comments to Bennett.

Butler and Denison looked from the tree. They both felt a little bit of relief.

It was shameful, but it wasn't more than when John Jenkins, a bright-eyed man, poured into the party with his friends. Hollenback and he met up and grabbed each others' arms, shaking vigorously, with smiles beaming across their faces.

Denison slowly rose and walked to the conclusion, "There is the solution."

The group. He glanced back over his shoulder and waved to Butler behind.

Wyoming's spirit is that! "Let's not lose it again dear friend!"

Butler smiled wide, nodding. Kicking his

He spiritedly rode to the cabin, his legs pressed into his mount's flanks. "Well, men," he declared, "let's get to the point!" He lifted one leg above the saddle and suddenly forgot all about his pains. He jumped from the saddle and slapped his mount on its rump. He rolled up his worn sleeves and marched through the men, stopping only for a pine knot at the fire. He swung it around the cabin, finally tucking it in a hole in the wall.

He said, grasping at one of the "small, but it will do for a beginning",

Take down the charred logs. The rest of the trees seem strong enough to withstand any future damage. You get to do that, while others get to go and cut trees to make a stockade to welcome Indian Butler, if he is foolish enough to return. He said that it was, while looking at Hollenback, Jenkins, and asking them if they could suggest a better stockade.

Both of them replied, "No," "all is razed and burnt that we have,"

encountered."

Denison said, "So be it," and grabbed an axe before heading to the tree.

line. "We'll do what we can, but I promise you that soon we will erect a new fort against these painted rats!"

The huzzas are energized and ring!

out. Wyoming was alive again that night, its spirit beating through men's veins promising it would not fall again.

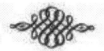

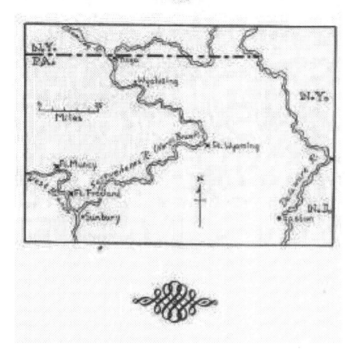

Chapter Four

Zebulon Butler jumped out of the stockade half-full and quickly mounted his horse. The sound of the north's lively shots made his spine tingle. He glanced back and saw his men quickly drop their axes. They grabbed their shot bags, powderhorns, bags, and firelocks. They ran along the road quickly, each checking their weapons and knowing that they would be ready to fire within seconds.

They were relieved to find that the shots decreased as they got closer to the target.

disturbance. Butler remembered an earlier alarm. Although it was less active, it had chased away quite a few feathered or painted heads within the tree line. The threat was growing, however. The threat was growing, and the Indians were coming back in greater numbers.

He rode down to the small group of men huddled in a clearing and then he stopped.

He scanned the tree line intently, paying attention to what was happening. He slowed his mount and pulled out a gun from his belt. He shouted at the men, "Where are they?".

Robert Carr replied, "They've scattered again," lowering his voice.

His eye was the spyglass. Carr said, "Don't know their numbers, but they fired one volley, and scampered away!" He nodded towards the man in front of him.

He was looking up at Butler as he inspected a new hole in his hunting.

shirt. The man replied, "They almost got me," but "I've still got mine, thank God for that!"

Butler nodded and turned to acknowledge the man at the fort.

They will rush to you. He said, "Slow down Lord." "They have scattered again."

Lord Butler was overcome by the sight of his father, tall in the sky.

saddle. His face was full of pride, regardless of what the others thought. The teenager was slightly relieved but anxious to have the chance to be as brave as his father. He walked a few feet to the front, holding his rifle in his hands. He looked over the entire tree line and nodded to his father as he surveyed the other men around him.

Butler, looking up at the trees, said "Yes, we must scout it."

setting sun. "But don't go far, all must retreat to the fort when it sets. To be out here unprotected, is the greatest folly and I will not have any of it." He said, cutting off the men's protests. He wished everyone understood the importance of building forts before trying to gather the cattle and other livestock that were wandering through the forest. These men wouldn't be ordered. He knew that they had to be led. He was not haunted by the horror of the Battle of Wyoming, but he continued to think in the New England ideal of democracy.

He turned a bitter eye at Captain William Hooker Smith commander

The remains of the Twenty Fourth Connecticut Militia Regiment were seen rushing up, huffing, and trailing their muskets behind them.

Carr reported the news to his portly commander, "They've disappeared.".
Smith gasped. "Yes," Smith said. All foraging parties have returned to

The camp soon, it grows long." He looked up at Butler, realizing he had disregarded the colonel's headstrong orders.

Butler replied, "Very well," before turning his attention back to the regulars.

who he did command. "Captain Spalding, have your men, save those on scout return and continue their work. It is vital that the stockade is completed with all due haste. This is impossible due to the increasing frequency of the enemy. It is a wish that others would have the same insight.

Hooker Smith sweated. Hooker Smith rubbed his sweating brow.

to do? All the things these men had in the world were buried in the ashes. They were determined to save everything they could. Who could blame them? He said "Yes," and all who can should support Captain Spalding's men. It is, as the Colonel states, of great importance.

Knowing his feelings, Butler gave Smith a gentle bow of the head.

He declared affirmation to be the best that he could offer at this time. The group turned back and walked back to camp, watching out for any bushes or tree lines. In the distance, thunder clouds roared. In the darkness, lightning flashed from the forks. The colonel's words were echoed in the minds of the militiamen with each closing boom.

Colonel Butler was struck by the affirming glances he received from the

He stood in ranks and looked back at the angry flashes that lit up the dark. He mumbled under his breath, "Thank you Providence," Even if his words of warning were ineffective, he knew that nature's warnings rang in men's souls and hearts. Wyoming remained at the knife's edge.

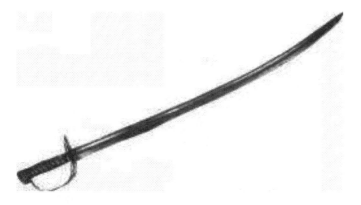

Chapter Five

Colonel Butler leaned back on his badly repaired chair. He leaned back in his chair, heeding its warning. He was captivated by the flickering light from the pine knot that had been tucked between the logs of his cabin's walls. He looked down at the paper before him and listened to the sounds of soldiers making the stockade from firelight outside. He paused to wonder if providence was at work when he heard the thunderous roar of a storm rolling through the air. He bowed his head and said a quick prayer before he opened his eyes to see the paper.

He slowly took his quill and dipped it in an ink well.

Maple bark ink was used to begin writing:
"Camp Westmoreland August 5, 1778"

The most honorable Colonel Hartley

Fort Augusta, Sunbury,
Yesterday, I arrived with approximately sixty Continental.

About forty militia and troops. Yesterday we found two small Indian groups, fired at them and found two more today. It is not known how many there are. Your honor may consider it appropriate to send some troops under your command up the river as far as this place or as far as you think is proper. I believe it will be a way of stopping the savages killing and robbing these frontiers inhabitants.

Colonel Butler,
commanding, Camp Westmoreland"

He quickly folded the paper after he had put the quill down. Hastily

He sealed it as best he could and called Captain Carr over to his side.

Half-opening the door to the cabin creaked open. Carr

He shuffled through the book, taking off his hat.

"As Mr. Goss and you have so graciously offered to run,

"Dispatches between I and Colonel Hartley. Here is the first," he stated, giving him the letter.

Carr grabbed the item immediately and carefully placed it in his bag

He carries a haversack over his shoulder.

Butler stated, "Be always mindful of your surroundings." "You are aware of your surroundings."

These cunning savages are a great example of their Tory brethren. As a seafarer as you were once, I am confident in your ability to navigate any storm. But this storm is unpredictable. These dispatches should not be lost under the enemy's eye, or you, my dear man, or Goss. So be very careful and act quickly.

Carr said "Yes sir," bowing slightly. "We shall depart

directly."

"I have instructed Captain Spalding that you each receive a brace pistols."

Butler stated that they have the best rifles available." "See him before your depart."

Carr nodded and disappeared into the shadows outside the door. It was

crept closed after him.

Butler rose from his seat and began to walk around, contemplating their possibilities.

He was unsure if he hadn't sent two men to their deaths. He was overcome by visions of the battle, which caused him to bow his head and clasp his hands behind his back. He closed his eyes to block the flashes of faces and thoughts that were coming into his mind. He would never again see the faces. Faces he had ordered. "No, my children!" After a moment of agony and reflection, he shouted "No!" He rode back along the battle line, beseeching his men not to surrender to the terrible onslaught. He was certain of his words, and he didn't hesitate to hold on for a few more shots. O cruel hand of fate! Why must these good men die and suffer to make Providence's hand known in this wild wilderness? Why? Why? He was unable to stop his anguish and began speaking out loudly, choking the words down so that no one would hear.

Lord opened the door and saw his son. Lord

He looked around for a moment, trying to find the ghosts his father had spoken to, but he couldn't find them. He concluded that they were in his father's mind. Ghosts lived in the mind and soul.

Butler stated, "I have sent Captain Carr to Fort Augusta"

He noticed his son staring out of the corner his eyes. "Command can weigh heavily on a man's mind, son. Oh, the suffering General Washington must endure in this beleaguered state of his soul!" These feelings are not to be allowed to cloud your judgment. They will bring you down, so don't dwell too long on them.

Lord replied, "Yes, Father." Slowly, he sat down in a trencher that he had held.

There was plenty of food on the table. It was overflowing with fresh and colorful beef, mutton and corn. "You must eat as everyone else has. With the strays being gathered and all, food is plentiful again. We had every right to return. Thanks to the enemy's oversight, the fields are abundant and there will be a good harvest. Carr and Goss are not to be worried about. I made sure they were armed and ready to go when they left. If they do encounter any savages, it was me who did so. My scout brought five sheep and two bullocks alone!

Butler ran his fingers through his hair and was suddenly embarrassed. A

He thought to himself that a commander should not dwell too much on the past but must learn from its failures and gain strength from its victories.

He sat down, hoped for the feast, and dug into the bounty.

It helped to ease some of his anxiety. He said, "Hartley's entire Regiment has been ordered up here," and he ate a lot, realizing how hungry he was. "Brodhead is already at the West Branch. My boy, spirit is what all of us possess, despite our differences. We should not be suspicious of West Branch settlements despite the destruction of Charleston and Judea settlements and the fact that they are mostly from Pennsylvania and Jerseys. There is a greater enemy than us all at the moment and he must be defeated if we want to have anything. Hartley was one of those men who shared the same sentiment. Hartley drank a large amount of rum from a wooden mug. "Ah, let's start a distillery as soon as possible after we finish the fort. A man must drink!"

Lord stated, "We have three full hogsheads," "We must..."

not thirst."

Nathan Denison was now a better man as the door creaked once more. He moved across the room holding his own corn and meat trencher. He said, "The corn is a little green, but it's good, by jingo!" and he plopped down on a blanket near the hearth. He also took a big gulp from his noggin. "I think we will be fine Zebulon. The longer we stay, I believe things are looking better."

Butler raised his toasty finger to say, "Huzzato that Nathan!" He thought silently about the small militia groups that had taken over the task of raising the fort. He thought about the complaints of some opportunistic people who took what little property was left after the battle. He was aware that all depended on the post being maintained, at least until harvest. To ensure their success, things must change. It was essential for the health of children's stomachs. It was essential for widows. It was vital for future generations.

Not at all. Let those who oppose change the course of events.

Order is a curse. He heard the cries of both the dead and the living in his head and was beseeched by them. He knew that all men of good judgment would follow his example. He only hoped that the actions he had now chosen would not be a hindrance to the independent spirit he loved. He took another long drink and fought against the new thought. They needed discipline to survive. He prayed that it would strengthen their resolve rather than weaken it. The Six Nations warriors were all around him, and he knew this. They were there. They were terrifying to him and they could only be defeated by a well-organized force.

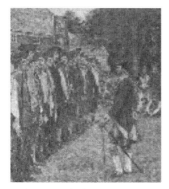

Chapter Six

Captain Spalding woke up with a jolt right before dawn. His mind was still cluttered with thoughts that he had carried all night. It was a difficult night of sleep. His brow was already wet. He looked around at the men scattered about him, and noticed that the humid air was still stagnant. The men lay in every possible position in the crowded stockade. Some were covered with blankets while others were covered with furs or deerskins, but the majority of them were on the hard, bare earth.

He stretched out and gazed out through a loophole.

It. Nothing was found outside of the walls. He wiped the sleep from his eyes and stumbled to the stockade's entrance, its half-finished gate tucked next to him. The sentry stood up and saluted the lone man.

He said, "No need for such Stephens," and placed his hand on the item.

Man's shoulder, "too soon in the morning."

Stephens said, "Fine sir," over the sound of many snores. A few

Many people made snorts and lip smacks, which filled the air with disgusting sounds of swallowing.

Spalding stated, "They sleep hard", and "as they live."

He turned his head to the nearest fire place and looked at his eyes. He slung his bag around his chest and pulled out a small piece of his brain. Stephens asked, "Is there any coffee inside that pot?".

He said, "Should it be, but it has been sitting all night," "Do you want?"

You can make it new?

Stephens' swelling lip was the first thing he noticed. He was captivated by the fight between him and Moses Brown last night.

Stephens was struck by his stare. Stephens replied, "Yes," but he suggested, "But you should see Moses' eye!" He turned again and looked at the green beyond the gate and the trees. He said, "But at the very most, I don't blame him." "A good half-dozen left the fort last evening, playing what mischief whom is to know?" He bowed his heads, thinking he might be out of line but someone had got to say something. "Someone returned, neglecting my challenge and mocking me for asking for parole. It's hell for Moses, who is not allowed to look around his cabin while others can freely." He shrugged. We all felt the effects of his curses and threats to quit the ranks when his enlistment ends in just a few weeks. "I couldn't contain my anger.

Spalding sat still, letting Stephens calm his conscience.

His words. He was upset to see his close friends, who had been through so much over the past two years, come to blows. Wyoming was a hotbed of tension. This fact kept him awake at night.

Stephens turned to face the captain and said "Still," "It was just a..."

soldier's fight. Given the hardships we have endured, I would hope that no charges will be filed. After the horrors of Forty Fort, Moses had to leave his infant sons and wife back at Fort Penn. Fort Penn offers them much charity, but it is hard to predict how long. It is a great way to test his nerves.

Spalding nodded at Stephen for his defense of him friend, even after the fact.

There were many harsh words and blows exchanged between them last night. Their friendship, which spanned from Millstone, New Jersey to Brandywine and Valley Forge, was unbreakable. Their brotherhood gave him strength.

Stephens said, "It's not like either of us is fist-bullies." Stephens said, "You of

All people need to know this, as we both have faithfully served you through this terrible tragedy, the Revolutionary War."

Spalding's eyes lit up at the mention of the new word.

war. It was something he had heard before, and he liked its sounding since it sounded real. He suppressed a smile at thinking of the small-framed man who considered himself to be a bully. He quickly made his decision and answered the questions that had been bothering him throughout the night. He sighed and said, "Yes, I know my good friend, and all of you have contributed should never be forgotten, by the this, or future generations," "If Moses feels it is necessary to leave the ranks after the expiration date of enlistment. It is yours and his.

Stephens stated, "You are correct of course." "Thank you, my family!"

It is safe in Connecticut. He is safe in Connecticut. He raised his rifle and gazed at the dawn light, only to lower it to the sound of distant laughter, followed by whoops of triumph in English-Yankee English.

He shook his head and said: "Something must happen, sir.

due respect."

Spalding, rising from the fireside, said "I know." Back brushing

He tied his hair by his hands with a leather strip. He walked towards the cabin door, his eyes widening in deep thought. He pushed it aside and walked through the door unannounced.

Butler said "Captain Spalding", slowly rising from his hearth

He rubbed his freshly shaven forehead. Straightening up his worn clothes, he glanced over at Denison, who was also sitting by the fire. He said, "We were about to call you," and added that he was glad to see him up and about after yesterday's hard work. It was a great job. After this day, the fortifications will be completed. Then, we will see about a bigger, more powerful fort.

Spalding replied, "But as for morale or the general well-being of the community,"

It is the responsibility of all residents to do something. It is necessary to have the ability to rebuild our homes and communities. If we want to attract others back, it must be like that!

Butler replied, "Yes, yes, dear man," and cautioned that "you should not get into a

tizzy."

Spalding gasped in frustration and rolled his eyes. Denison

He took a deep inhale and held the clay pipe between his teeth for a while. A long trail of smoke was visible through his lips as he smiled. Butler pulled out a single paper from his pocket and smiled. He tossed it in the air and handed it to the captain.

Spalding lifted it to the greased paper window, and then read it.

He nodded his head affirmatively, He said, "It's just," and handed the paper to him.

Denison. Colonel, "Something had got to be done. I also see no other way.

Denison replied, "Oh, keep that, sir." "We spoke half the night.

We did and came to the same conclusion."

Spalding looked at the paper and shrugged.

Butler stated, "You must address the men with this new directive." "We must have them all assembled immediately." He grinned at the upsetting thought. "Have ya seen Captain Smith?"

"No sir. Very few people are astir after last evening."

"Well, we will see to it, let's have this for breakfast!" Butler said, carefully putting his hat on and leading the group through the door. They were greeted by few people in the early morning sunlight, except Stephens, who smiled at being relieved of guard duty and a few others, all carrying a pick-and-splol.

Butler called out to them, prompting them all to shout, "Here Captain Smith!"

Stop and turn your head to face him.

Smith stated, "We" are about "something which shall prove a".

pleasant surprise, fine sir."
Butler stated, "Yes, well, that's it, we all have some surprises this morn." "Beat the drum, and assemble your men. Are they all around?

Smith raised an eyebrow as he slowly looked around the stockade.

He raised his lower lip. He said, "Most, I suppose." "We are going to dig up the four-pounder!" It was wrapped tightly and buried at the end of battle to prevent the enemy from capturing it. It is buried in the exact spot I know!"

A short distance away another officer was listening and darted

He rubbed his right hand curiously towards them. "What? "What? He shook his head and asked "I wanted that damn thing brought up to Forty Fort in late battle and you buried?".

Butler stated, "Now, Jenkins, it was probably the best at that time." It was impossible to carry a carriage and a ball.

Jenkins asked, "Best for whom?" Jenkins asked, "Best for whom?"

It would have scared many of them. It is called thunder death. It was a foolish thing to do. You could have loaded it up with lead balls, stone, and such!

Butler stated, "Yes, but the past is history." "We can only learn."

From the past. Captain Smith, is that not right?

Smith looked wide-eyed at Jenkins as he ran away from them. The man's knowledge of Indians was undisputed. He had been their captive for several months and knew them well.

Butler replied, "Yes, now," "about your men."

Their attention was drawn to the gate by a sharp, slapping sound. Stephens slammed his arms and stared nervously at the colonel.

Butler replied, "Yes, my man. Have you anything to say?" "Have

not you been relieved?"

"Yes, sir," Stephens said, "But begging your pardon, sir." He

Captain Spalding was a subject of great anxiety.

Spalding said, "Go ahead Stephens," with a nod towards Colonel Butler.

"The other members of the militia, sir? they can range freely without regard

Stephens said that proper order and such is what Stephens was looking for, ignoring Smith's bitter gaze. He said, "But all that have been around in the night have returned," and he continued, "for now at least."

Butler: "Yes, that's right, we will soon see about it, we will,"

Answered, nodding to drummer.

A lively call was immediately made to the assembled men by the drum. Men rose.

Some grumbled, others less enthusiastically than others. But soon, they were all standing in a straight line in the cramped stockade.

Butler moved in front of them, with his hands tightly clasped behind him.

He looked at every part of the regal commander. He looked at each man. Others shook their heads, while others ignored him.

"What are you about?" A voice spoke from behind him. "Ye are not Washington."

Butler looked in the direction of the insult with his eyes wide open, glaring back at him.

With anger. He yelled "Officers!" and said, "See to your men, be smart!" My fine lads are not a rabble now! Things are about to change, damnit! Attention to Orders!" He marched up to Captain Spalding and waved at him to read the letter aloud.

Spalding cleared his throat and waited impatiently for the grumbles

to die.

Butler followed him, ready to tie the knot.

Spalding raised the paper and began to speak:

"Detachment orders, Camp Westmoreland August 7, 1778"

"Our current situation seems rather dangerous and alarming.

Our entire interest and the remaining prospects of our crops depend on us maintaining the Post and taking possession of the country. Therefore, everyone will feel the strongest possible tie to the defense of the place and be held responsible for doing his best against the common enemy. It is impossible to make ourselves powerful in any way without maintaining order and discipline. Therefore, the martial law must be strictly observed by all militia members and those who are part of the Colonel Butler detachment.

"The pernicious practice to walk about in small groups, and

It is dangerous to the good order and unsafe for the individual to be absent without leave. The Colonel is concerned about the allegations that evil people have been taking advantage of private property and making it waste. He forbids the killing of sheep, swine, or poultry, as well as any other way of injuring the interest of any man.

"For [the] Future the Guard is to be relieved at 6 o'clock in The

Morning, and the roll is to be called twice daily: morning and night. Officers will be especially vigilant to ensure that the order is followed. Non-commissioned officers are required to enforce the order on soldiers and provide early information about any breaches. All who are found guilty in breach of this order could face the harshest consequences.

      Officers of the Day-This-Day, Lieutenant Gore and Lieutenant Pierce; Tomorrow, Lieutenant Pierce."

      Spalding lowered the letter and stood suddenly at Spalding's attention.

He regained his military bearing. He noticed a sudden change in the men's stances. Butler's piercing eyes saw that Butler was removing the days of lack of discipline. They could see that he meant everything.

      Spalding stepped back and gave way to the wall of the cabin.

In the crowded stockade. Butler moved forwards without muttering a single word. He didn't care if his orders said it all. He would now stand and allow them to take it in under his steely eyes.

      His heart was interrupted by a scream that echoed through the woods to his north.

stance. It faded at first, only to be re-echoed in a different direction but it was closer. Each time the war cries were heard, they echoed in every direction. But none at once and only after each previous one had ended. They stood firm but all looked out from the corner of their eyes at the green hills where the cries were echoing. Their hard eyes were filled with worry, but they held firm under the watchful eye of their commander. They would not move again, and that is when they were given orders.

The only man at the gate was the sentry. He paced nervously around.

He raised his rifle towards one of the cries, and then he stopped. He became more upset as they got closer. He looked back at the stockade and saw his frozen comrades. Nobody said a word. He was not helped by anyone.

He heard a close cry just to his left, above a small knoll. He raised

He fired his gun and cursed the noise that made his spine tingle. He yelled, "Shut up murdering savages!" and scanned the stockade anxiously. Nobody moved. He wondered aloud, "What has overcome all?" "The murdering devils have arrived!" Cannot you hear? ?"

Butler said, looking smartly and saying "Relieve this man immediately."

Walking towards the cabin. Smith, get to the cannon! He called out to his colleague before entering the cabin.

Spalding stated, "They are just playing their games." He stepped to the

men's fear and anxiety. "Just trying to scare us. They know that a feathered head will be receiving a ball, so you won't see it. All will be well if you follow your orders. Now officers, take control of your men.

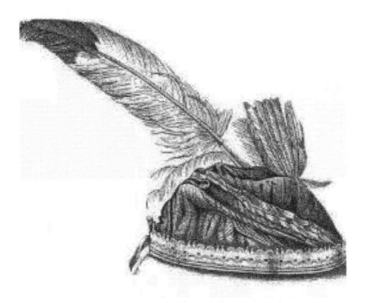

Chapter Seven

"Paxtang (Pennsylvania, July 12, 1778

Supreme Executive Council of Pennsylvania

Philadelphia
"I am reluctant to write this letter, but I know it must be.

Give pain to any man with a sense of humor. On Wednesday, July 8, I had to leave Sunbury and my entire property. Never in my entire life have I seen such distress. The roads and river were clogged with people, women and children fleeing for their lives. Many had no property and many left behind the most important part. The Northumberland County has been broken up. Col. Samuel Hunter remained but he did his best to rally the people and make a stand against the enemy. He was left with only a handful of men to rely on. Wyoming has been abandoned. There was not one family left between Wyoming and

Sunbury when my departure. This place is filled with panic and fear. Many have moved out of the township, and almost everyone thinks of a place that offers greater security.

"For God's sake, for the sake of our country-let Colonel Hunter

Sunbury to be strengthened. If you are unable to do more, send him only one company. Charity should be offered to the many poor and displaced persons who clog the banks of this river. These are people I don't used to love but now I most deeply sympathize with their suffering. "William Maclay"

The man sat at his desk, thinking, "Quite a letter indeed," said the man.

The same Colonel Hunter, who was mentioned in the lines, stood solemnly as Colonel Brodhead and his regiment marched out of Fort Augusta's gates to continue their trek towards Fort Pitt. He watched as the other regal men stood by him. General De Haas sat stoically, his thoughts apparently focused on other matters. He had sent small militia groups up the river to replace Brodhead's men. He was accompanied by a taller, more respectable man who looked at him with concern. General Potter, a hard-eyed man, sometimes turned his attention to one of the officers to offer some advice. He looked at General Potter, who was sitting behind a glass desk and observing them only once before turning his attention back to the soldiers at the gate. He admired the man at the window.

The polite refusal of both the generals to accept command was a sign of respect.

He listened to the words of gentlemen in his head as he turned away from the widow and stared at the papers on the desk before him. The full weight of command fell on his shoulders, even though he was a rank lower than the other high-ranking officers. He sighed and began to thumb through copies of other letters, begging the Continental Congress or anyone else to take action.

They had now acted. He sat there, confused to say the least.

Moreover, none of the pages could capture the despair that gripped the country. He was now compelled by General Washington to defend five hundred miles of frontier with only one regiment and promises to a thousand militiamen. He didn't hold his breath waiting for the militia. He was left with a small group of brave settlers and his two-hundred-man unit. It was impossible, but war made it possible and he did his best to make it work.

He stood up and looked out the window at Maclay's letter, as well as the wall that juts out to the east. His free hand rubbed his eyes, his eyes with a stiff continence. But he felt warm, mysterious, and deep as if surrounded by men his age. His muscular, but slightly pudgy frame filled the window. He was as tall as any Pennsylvania farmer's son, not as commanding and bold as George Washington or as bright and bold as General 'Mad' Anthony Wayne, but he was sincere and stern. He was a man of the people, as well as looking like them. His deeper nature was also evident. Men such as Washington, Wayne, and others recognized him and called him friend. This is no small feat, considering the high standards of these two great generals. While he was still taking a deep breath, he refused to let either of them down.

He turned and bit his lip before settling down in the chair.

Behind the desk. He quickly dipped a pen into ink and wrote a report to congress, verifying the reports of all others.

For a moment, his concentration was interrupted by a slight knock at the front door.

Moment, but he quickly recovered his thoughts and grumbled 'Enter' at the door.

The soldier entered the room smartly and waited for the others.

Before speaking, stop the pen from tracing across the paper. He said "Colonel Hartley", while watching him fold the paper and seal it with wax. "Your mount awaits, and the men are assembled for march."

Hartley motioned to his blue regimental uniform coat, "Very well," Hartley replied.

hanging by the door.

The soldier quickly grabbed the package and opened it.

Hartley carefully placed his finely cocked cap on his head, and he slid his arms into the hat.

On his head. "Yes Captain Walker, there is still much to do, I am afraid. We must get to Muncy's and Wallis' houses as soon as possible. "We must also strike at the heart and soul of the enemy."

Walker replied, "Yes sir," referring to the colonel's comment about needing to

Strike at the enemy's heart, echoing in his head. He thought about it. He couldn't think of a better man than the one before him to lead them.

Hartley said, "But one must look before they are to leap," Hartley continued.

He nodded his head. "Colonel Brodhead and his regiment may now feel more free to prey on the settlements. We must stop them from pursuing the frontier's fringes. We will show Indian Butler what we have for him, no matter how small our numbers.

Following the strong little, Walker bobbed his forehead in affirmation.

Get out of the way. He thought of the colonel's gleaming eyes and decided to do something. Washington and Congress had done a good thing by choosing this man to secure frontier. Few could compare to his zeal, determination and resolve.

Perhaps this nation can overcome with men like he.

You can overcome seemingly impossible odds to win victory over a distant tyrant and become independent. These men shined through the dark clouds of despair that hung over the newly formed nation. There is more to courage and zeal than mere zeal. It is something that can be paired with all the good things that are new to the world. As all things new, whether they are ideas or nations, it either possessed them or lost them.

The thing called spirit.

Chapter Eight

"Get after them!" "Get after them!" Colonel Hartley exhorted the men ahead of him. A few fleet-footed men ran after a blur of painted men, sprinting towards the tree line. Many of the men reloaded and fired at the painted devils quickly, but they vanished into the trees, appearing to melt into underbrush.

Hartley called the heads of "Captain-Lieutenant Sweeney!"

The men climbed atop his nervous mount. "Call the men back!" They are in for an ambush in the underbrush!

Sweeny gave the orders and waved back a disappointment

Squad of men. They turned around reluctantly cursing their bayoneted muzzles. They were almost taunted by their quick escapes and fleet-footed foe, who disappeared again and again under the incorrect fire of their muskets.

Hartley yelled, seemingly indifferent to their demands.

complaints.

General De Haas stated that "their complaints are valid."

Hartley could hear the sound. Hartley shook his head as he moved closer to Hartley's mount. He said, "Brodhead had that same problem, and some his men, along with the militia, do possess the rifle and the tomahawk.".

"The way they dart around only to disappear like a ghost intothe

Hartley looked down at his horse and said that forest is not uncanny." Hartley said, "Perhaps four legs with a swan shot into every cartridge box would even out the odds.".

De Haas grinned. The idea was a good one. He said, "Perhaps," Hartley's resilience impressed him, and perhaps Congress has chosen the right man to do the job. He pointed with his free hand to the river, saying, "Wallis' was only a mile away, upstream." He said, "They harass those who have braved dangers to return to harvest the crops." "There is not a single cabin left standing, but the fields remain unmowed."

Hartley stated that "They took it for themselves, believing they could get rid of the Susquehanna from us." They are regrettably wrong in that. They have unwittingly strengthened the resolve of good people, instead of weakening it."

De Haas said, "I hope so," while looking at the blackened spots.

There was a lot of ground where once stood cabins amid the ripening grain fields. It was a strange juxtaposition.

Hartley said, "Dreams of good lives and the hope for them lay in those ashes."

said. "We must do everything we can to help these people reclaim the land."

De Haas believed Congress had chosen the right man. But, it may not have been.

He had given him the wrong tools. Hartley's fine blue regimentals had white faces, which he admired. Many of them already displayed the hardships of frontier duty, with ripped cuffs and missing buttons. He noticed that some feet had moccasins, as well as durable buckskin britches or trousers. This made him realize that most people have switched from their torn linen to buckskin britches out of necessity. He also noted that the same was true for footwear. These men were mostly from Berks or Chester Counties and were farmers, traders, and merchants. They had spent too much time in Philadelphia's shadow. From the introductions of Fort Augusta's officers, he remembered the merriment of the ranks from Delaware, Maryland, and Virginia. But they all seemed to be of the same caliber. They were all of the same feather. He reminded himself that these were the tools they had been given. You have to make do.

The sight of English's huge green lot brought a smile to his eyes.

They had grass in front of them. Hartley waved Hartley with his column in the direction of it, and they were led down the trail to a large stone house. The stone haven was marked by charred timbers. Brodhead's men may have camped in these areas, as evidenced by the presence of embers and grass from fire pits all over the green.

From the partially-burned stone door, a spirited man ran

house, he lifted his hat off his head and smiled from ear to hear. The man said "My, My," bowing to De Haas, and looking around at the men behind. Hartley was the focus of his eyes. He said, "You, Colonel Hartley!" and extended his hand. "It is very grand to see you, and in command a fine lot if soldiers!"

> Hartley said, "Yes, Mr. Wallis. I presume," and he put his hand to his mouth.

He slowly eased out of the saddle. He brushed his regimental clean and looked around the house.

> Wallis declared, "Walls are three-foot thick all around." "Rifle

Every wall has slits. It was too hard to burn, even though the Indians tried. But it is still standing." He stood on the ground and stomped his feet. "And this is where my bones will rest, God save me!"

> Hartley extended his hand and said "Yes", Hartley said, extending his hand.

The man was a great example of grit. It suggested a deeper resolve in his character. Hartley said, "I heard that you are of Society of Friends," noticing the pistols hidden in his belt. It was strange for a Quaker to do this.

> Wallis looked at the pistols and patted one of them on their backs.

butt. "Some believe one way while others believe another. God does not judge men for protecting their property. We on the frontier, unlike others who live in safe cities, have a more practical view of the world.

> Hartley was familiar with many Quakers, as he hails from York.

The man's friendly demeanor was refreshing and very different to any other Quaker he knew, except Nathanial Greene. He quickly became friendly with the man. He is a Quaker who has common sense.

"Now, if you and General shall see fit grace my humble

"Adobe, I will have my sincere thanks," he smiled with a beaming smile.

De Haas stated, "Well, I must admit, it's good to be appreciated."

gracefully dismounting.

Hartley stated, "The day becomes late." Hartley said, "Sir. Take your leave."

He turned to his officers.

Wallis stated, "By all means I am sorry that I don't have more to offer."

Spreading his hand across the green grass. "But, sir. You are most welcomed by us all. Your fatigue camp should be set up exactly where Brodhead's was, and all around the green.

Hartley replied, "Very well." Hartley said, "Captains take control and dismiss the

column. For the evening, we will camp here. Put up a strong picket."

The men escaped from the ranks to get onto the grass at their feet.

officers' behest. The black man quickly appeared from the house and directed the men with a warm smile towards the nearest spring.

Hartley noticed that the man was looking at him for a second until Wallis.

He ushered him in the door. He mused about another peculiarity of a Quaker: his ownership of his fellow man. Evidently, this man was able to adapt to his environment and made do. De Haas didn't seem to have any reservations about the man, and his resilience was refreshing. When Wallis offered him a fine cup of rum, he subdued all his fears. He finished the rum and settled down on the bench at the table.

One Quaker had a lot of wealth that he didn't have at the time.

He was a master of the area and would fight the devil to gain the knowledge he needed to complete his mission. He smiled wide and slapped the mug onto the table. He said, "Now, tell me, fine sir," and turned his attention to his host. "Everything about the land's nature and lay."

Wallis was thrilled to see suspicion melt when his eyes lit up at the invitation.

From the officer's eyes. His vibrant tongue was full of praises for the colonel, his regiment, Colonel Brodhead, the militia and General De Haas. He disarms them more and more with charm, before giving a detailed summary of everything he knew about the area, he being the largest landowner.

Soon, a lively murmur rose up from the green plain. Fires flittered

The air was filled with the scents of fresh-roasted beef, especially for men by the black man. Other men stood guard at every turn, watching and alert, along the slight rise in ground around the green and riverbank below. The men were not as comfortable as they thought, but the dreadful realization that their enemy was always at hand pushed them to think. They knew that somewhere in the darkness of the night, many eyes were watching their camp. Perhaps they were waiting for the dark shadows to strike and take their lives. Every rustle in a brush was given due attention. A suspicious eye paid attention to every hoot of an Owl.

Dover, Philadelphia and Richmond were all considered worlds.

These men were taken away, but they remained true to their duties.

Their honor demanded it.

Chapter Nine

Colonel Hartley looked at the huge elm in front of him. He paced around the elm, thinking it must be at least twenty feet in diameter. It alone could make a beautiful home. He looked around at the other trees and sighed. He mumbled under his breath, "What wealth lies in this virgin land." He ran his hands along the rough bark, reminiscing about the towering white pines and hemlocks that he had seen between Wallis and Sunbury. The Navy has won so many prizes! He saw masts for future ships every time he looked at the straight and fine pines. He was flooded with images of the fields full of lush grain. These mountains were rich in fertile and rich soil. His imagination was boggled by the fact that timber alone was enough to make so many homes. The land stretched for miles and each acre was more valuable than the last. He thought, "What a wonderful time to be alive!" It was a privilege to live and breathe at its beginning. This is the beginning of a new nation! This is the beginning of the new American Nation!

"Colonel," a voice calling from the tree.

He said slowly, removing his hand from the bark.

After straightening his clothes he took a few steps to the tree.

Standing by the tree's side, the man raised his eyes to the sky.

"Fine timber, many miles of it!" Wow!

Hartley replied, "Yes Captain Walker," "I have noticed."

Walker stated that there was something of God in all the things. Walker said, "And now he

he has helped his children prosper in its bounty. These times offer more. It makes a man feel small, and his complaints insignificant when compared to the beauty of it all.

Hartley stated, "Yes, I agree," and he looked towards a sharp.

A crackling sound was heard just above the ridge in front of them. It was followed by a huge crash.

Walker stated, "The harvest is beginning." Walker said, "Even if it's just for a while."

We must resist the heathens of the forest, and all those who would oppose God's will. It is a new fort.

Hartley nodded his head and walked towards the noise, "You're

He asked, "Are you already felling trees?" "We have just chosen a spot for the fort last night."

Walker stated, "Haste makes waste." "We won't let you down sir.

or our country."

Hartley looked at Hartley and said, "No, I don't think you will, nor the men."

The threadbare man. The bush had played havoc with their clothes, but not their spirit. The bush, their fleeting foe and only a faint aspirational, would flash about from time to time to make his presence felt, mocking and teasing them. It seemed to have no effect on their resolve. All his men saw determination.

He was determined and had a new, shinny American spirit. He felt

It made him feel hollow and made it difficult to see his potential as a leader. He had been exposed to the trials of the Canadian Campaign, and the battles surrounding Philadelphia. This enemy was different and more difficult to find. He slipped right through your fingers just as you thought you had him under your control. Every shadow, tree, and bush proved to be his haven. He struck at the most inopportune times, stealing a scalp, and then disappearing once more. Reports of new depredations were already coming in. It seemed futile to assign soldiers and militiamen for every party going to harvest a crop. There had to be more than defensive actions. He thought that one must strike the devils at their hearts, in their hideout, but he said it louder.

Walker stated, "I couldn't agree more.".
Colonel Hartley admitted, slightly embarrassed, that "Yes", but "first things first."

He glanced over his shoulder at the vast camp surrounding Wallis' stone home. They need to strike in large numbers, I fear.

Wyoming has shown us this, if not more.

Walker stated, "But they will not leave the fort once they strike like they did in Wyoming." "And I guarantee you it will be a strong fort when it's done."

Hartley stated, "I have no doubts, my good man.".
Walker began his march to the location of the new fort.

Show his commander the work that had been done. The entire area of the fort was free from scrub brush, and surveyors marked its outline.

Already, a few logs were in place and rising high into the sky with their

Pointed tops He slowed down with a grunt to his rear. Hartley was cursing Hartley's stump as he turned his head to examine his broken stockings and battered leg. The wound was drenched in blood.

Walker stated, "Leggings must be a necessity in this country." He was walking back

to him.

Hartley replied, "No, no," regaining his composure. He felt belittled

His torn stocking was visible in the faces of the ragged soldiers. He chuckled and said, "I'm fine, and you are correct, I need a pair of good buckskin leggings." "Damn frontier will take me yet, I fear."

Walker quickly turned around and shook his head.

He waved a few salutes at him. He said, "No need for such." "Not when a man works, anyway."

Hartley also waved the doffed caps. Hartley said, "The Captain is right."

said. "Be smart about what you do." He saw the men struggle under the massive logs. Even the massive oxen that pulled the logs struggled to lift their weight. The fort would be strong if the logs were laid with such care. He felt his heart beat faster as he watched the energetic workers. Each man worked hard, giving everything he had. These men merited the same effort and dedication from their leaders.

He moved slowly, taking care to keep clear of men and walking wide.

They are all of them. He was soon seated next to another officer, admiring the work as much as he did.

General De Haas stated, "A fine bunch of men indeed." He raised an awareness about the importance of this statement.

Hartley's eyebrow. "With such spirited men, I believe Congress has ordered the

These parts are a huge help. They will do the job."
Hartley replied.

De Haas retorted, pointing his riding crop at small bodies of water.

Men were placed at different points around the area. He called out to the closest group, "Look lively!" "Those devils, you know! They are cunning!" The men nodded and pointed to the group of horses strung by ropes heading towards them. They called the parole. They received an immediate countersign. The horses and men ran quickly past the sentries, heading straight for the officers.

De Haas asked, "What's that bugger about?" Notice a silver?

He added a strand to the shirt of his black hunting shirt by attaching it to his shoulder.

"Oh my God, isn't Carberry your man in the lead?"

Hartley answered, "Yes sir," and he took a few steps towards the man. He said, "Lieutenant Carberry", and greeted him.

Carberry raised a quick hand and touched the brim of his hat.

He donned a hat and steered a horse full-sided towards the officers. He reported that "this is fine stock!" and he extended his hand to the five other horses. "It is so good that we got them before the savages took them. They are, as I said, fine."

Hartley stated, while pacing about the horses, "Yes, they're," before halting.

Sometimes to run a hand down their legs. He said, "Fine horseflesh", and nodded to General De Haas.

De Haas: "In the current state of things they're yours to do what you want."

said. "I'm sure they have been lost by their owners."

Hartley stated, "This is very fine." "Lieutenant Carberry, my

"Good man, I have already written to headquarters asking permission for the raising of a company horse." He smiled and looked up at the horse's legs. "And I believe I have found Captain Carberry, the commander of that company."

Carberry's eyes lit up when he announced his instantaneous.

promotion. He said, "I would be honored sir." "Very honored! "I must say, sir!"

Hartley stated, "The honor is all mine Captain." "Saddles and

Along with sabers, holsters and sabers should be available. My good friend, now you need to erect a stable and collect more horses. Choose your men from the group, I'm sure you have men who are up to the task. You can rely on my experience and that of your men to help you with training. You will surely be up to the challenge.

De Haas stated, "We have to make do with what is available here." Your colonel is correct; these rats need four legs to be caught once they have reached full trot. They don't stand up and fight with their bloody-backed friends. They should try to outrun us now!

"Huzza!" Carberry, along with a few other men, shouted.

The general raised his head and waved his hand. The spirited

Many eyes looked around the fort at the exchange of words. They were accompanied by a pair of sluggish eyes that slowly walked towards them.

Hartley turned his head and asked: "Who is that crestfallen chap?"

towards De Haas.

The general declared, "Peter Smith." "Most unfortunate chap, indeed. His wagon, which contained his wife and their family, was driven by William King and some other unlucky souls to an Indian ambuscade in Plum tree thicket on Lycoming Creek. A massacre occurred. He and a few others escaped. It happened just before Wyoming's massacre. "He has been through a lot, but he has persevered." De Haas stopped speaking, noting the sad face within earshot. He reached out to help the sad soul.

> Smith nodded his head slowly, "General," he said. He shook his head.

He turned his attention to Hartley.

> Hartley observed Carberry's men lead the horses Carberry led. Hartley watched Hartley closely.

away. The sorrowful man's eyes were filled with recognition and he said he would release all or any of the animals to him. His eyes were still dull and stoic. Hartley extended his hand.

> Smith looked at Hartley and said, "You must be Hartley." "I

mean Colonel Hartley, don't mean no disrespect."

> Hartley replied, "Oh no, my dear one," and "none taken."

> Smith nodded and slowly let go of Hartley's grip. He rubbed his chin and gazed at the clearing ground and the rising logs in the fort. He said, "Not wasting any time, I see." "That's good. "I want to thank the soldiers for sharing their medicines and stores with these people. It is greatly appreciated by all of us, I assure.

> Hartley replied, "Yes," Hartley said, "I wish I had more." There are plenty of supplies

Although I am exhausted, I have sent an express to Council of War asking for more supplies, particularly medicine, to Coxe's Town. There I will see that it is forwarded to here, where it is most urgently needed.

Smith replied, "Well, I thank You Once Again, Fine Sir." Smith gazed.

He lowered his head to the ground, appearing to take in the words of the colonel and then contemplate his next words. He said, "If'n it won't be too trouble," and looked down at Wallis' house. "Some people have claimed that you send out soldiers to guard us as we go to the fields."

"Yes, we are."
"I have plenty of grain that needs to be reaped, cradled and enjoyed by my."

Just west of the Loyalstock is where Bull Run flows to the creek. Young Brady, Van Ness, as well as others, have pledged their support. However, it would be better for all if we had soldiers around us while we worked.

"No problem, my dear man, I will see to it personally."

Smith pointed to a group settlers who were following the trail.

The fort. The tall, muscular man leading the men wore a fine red stock that flowed across his shoulders. He kept his rifle close to his chest and was always ready for action, even when they entered the camp. His bright smile and cheerful disposition made him stand out from his more serious-faced peers.

Smith said "That there's James Brady," noticing Hartley and the General's stares at Smith's crimson-haired man. Smith said, "Yes, his brother Sam and father John are great Indian fighters. They have a certain air about their lives. James is the youngest. John is the oldest. However, they all carry the rank of captain. People around here call them all captains, but don't care what titles the proper people give them. The whole bunch of them are brave and fierce. John, Sam, his son, and the less-known John are fighting in Philadelphia. Proudly to call them friends, each and every one of them, I am at this." Smith then turned and trudged away, almost dragging his own beaten up firelock behind.

"Odd fellow," Hartley said. Hartley said, "But such are the rigors war."

Play on the souls of some men."

"Yes, poor fellow," De Haas added. "The people haven't

recovered. It is very confusing, disorienting, and distracting. When I return to York, I will do my best to ensure that you receive all assistance as soon as possible.

Hartley didn't say anything, his eyes were fixed on Smith, who was already speaking.

Wallis was most sincere to him as he sat on the ridge. He felt terrible for Wallis, but he also felt a sense of his own nature. The man was possessed by something hard, a hardness that twisted a man's beliefs. These men should be monitored, as sorrow and hardship can erode a man's loyalty from his rightful moorings. He observed them both in animated conversation, Wallis' hands rising and falling in great sweeping movements, only to be interrupted by Smith who seemed to have recovered from his sleepy state for the moment, with his arms still flying as animated.

Hartley stated, "What to do is be a bird and listen to what's being said."

under his breath.

De Haas stated, "Yes," but "we must do with the tools."

"Provided." He raised an eyebrow, appearing to agree with the Colonel's instinctive warning.

Both of them looked up at the rising logs in the fort and the downfall.

The ridge that leads to Wallis' home is within easy reach of the new fort. Each officer listened to his arguments and insisted that the fort should be built on his property. They had both stood in his beautiful house and noticed that while many people lost their belongings, only a few of his items were missing. They had enjoyed fine meals and drank from his pewter mugs. It was clear that the Indians and Tories would have had to take all of it. It remained.

De Haas stated, "He does share General Washington's confidence."

Hartley is already feeling anxious. "He seems to have a sincere affection for you, so he cannot be all bad."

"Yes, but sometimes things don't always turn out as expected, especially for men."

There is always an opportunity. Hartley stated that such a flag waved over the victorious man. "But, as you said, it is necessary to make do with what tools we have. So here Fort Muncy will stand. It is midway between Great Island and Bald Eagle Mountain, so it's the best spot.

The men looked at one another and nodded, before chasing each other away.

They felt a sense of hope in the face the despair that now surrounds them. Their promise remained with the people. For the moment, a deal could be made with Satan. He could prove fatal to their cause, but woe to him.

Woe indeed.

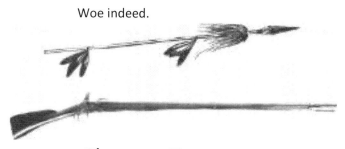

Chapter Ten

James Brady extended his arms and walked out of the cabin door with his rifle. He squinted as he watched the fog rise in the face the rising sun. He scanned the fields through breaks in the fog. The previous day's work had brought forth the wheat sheaves. He thought that one more day of good harvest would bring the harvest to an end. He thought for a while about Peter Smith's departure, which he and three others made last night out of some trivial excuse. It was quite odd, considering he owned all the fields. He argued that we all must keep together in such times. These crops would provide food for all of them in the coming winter.

A voice said, "You going to eat some victuals? Or not?"

from the cabin door.

He turned to see an elderly man with a spoon in his hand. "I'll

Van Ness, be there shortly," he said to his side.

"I wouldn't be out there with that soup if I were you, alone.

Van Ness sighed and turned back to the door. Van Ness said, "You better get moving, got seventeen other to feed, you know, one hungryer than the next, after seeing how all of you worked like the devil yesterday."

"I'll be there, old man. Just want to look around a little."

"There's nothing more than the devil in that fog!"

"Then, the devil will get one."

"And you the tomahawk!"
Brady turned and looked at the disgruntled elderly man. He said, "I'm coming to shut you up!" He took his rifle and checked the flint, before returning to his cabin. Two more soldiers appeared at the doorway, each one hungrily consuming their wooden noggins.

"Oh, it just feels so much better having all the soldiers here.

Eight of you," Brady laughed as he passed them. After you've finished filling your gizzards, best tend to your arms."

Both men nodded even though they were both corporals. The man spoke with the confidence of someone who is used to being followed. They thought it was no surprise that he was called captain by the other men.

One of them said, between bites, "You do your work," and "We'll do it."

ours."
Brady said, "I hope so," to the stunned man.

"Damn, if you people around these parts don't have eyes like hawks!"

"And ears like elephants!" said the other soldier. "If there were anything in the fog, you would know it," the other soldier said. You are indeed a difficult lot.

Brady stated, "Have-to-be, keeps our hair where its supposed to be,"

He shook one of his long red hairs back over his shoulder. He sat down on a stool near the hearth and pulled out a long, black iron swivel with a poker. He grabbed the spoon from the old man standing beside him and scooped out a large portion of the stew into his wooden noggin. Some of the stew spilled onto the floor.

"Tarnation!" The old man said, "There's plenty, we ain't got."

They were enough to feed the hogs!" He kicked them back into the fire. They smilked.

Brady stated, "Ain't no hogs around, anyhow." "Injuns got 'em all!"

They did it all, except for one big red-headed one.

"Day ain't over yet. But if they are brazen enough to attempt, I'll be

I'll make them pay a lot for this scalp. They'll still have a bright red lock to help them navigate the dark night if they manage.

"Ain't nothing to have fun about!" You cantankerous young rowdy! Get on with your work. We can get out of this mess quicker if we do it sooner. It gives me the willies, with all that fog and all."

Brady laughed and grabbed a rum sachet. He said, "Old man's right."

He sat up on the stool and took a big gulp of the Rum. "Daylight's burning! He rose high after consuming a few more spoonfuls of stew. He ignored the spoon and the noggin on the ground, and marched through the front door clutching his rifle like his best friend.

There were a few protest grunts, but most of them fled the door.

Behind the large, red-haired man. Four men reached out to grab the cradles that were next to the house, and he pointed them towards him.

"Well, it's all about you four cradling while we others head down to

The field yonder, and finish the last day of reaping. Brady said, "Ye soldiers, see about sentry.".

Three soldiers were separated from their militia counterparts and taken to the streets.

They went about their business. Brady was followed by the other soldiers and the harvesters down a steep hill to a field beneath the cabin.

They ran to the spot on the field from the previous day's.

work. Brady was the most disgusted as they sat around their rifles in front of a tree after gazing nervously around the fog.

He said, while he was holding his weapon.

Place your feet a few feet from the ground. "Spread 'em out."

He looked at them with wide eyes and then into the fog. One of them stated, "Capt'n, you can do whatever you want, but we's wants'em up, round the tree, so that we can get at them more easily if necessary," while the other took their scythes, and began to work.

Brady looked at his watch, realizing that his words were lost on the ears of his audience.

He was eager to finish his work and get off the field. He reached for a scythe and stared at the soldier who was standing next to him. He called out to the corporal, who was looking around at the area and seemed to be wondering where to put his men. He looked at the soldier in front of him again. He took the hint and marched slowly into the fog to the ridge, without any encouragement from his corporal. In these parts, the word of the frontier captain held true, at least in the art and practice of Indian fighting.

"The rest will spread out and form picket lines," said the

According to corporal, Brady was more important than his men. His men were able to see the harvesters and trees around them, regardless of their distance.

Brady sat watching, until everyone gave their approval. He said, "That'll do. Now we'll put back our heads to it while the sun's still hidden in the fog," and immediately began swinging his scythe through the wheat in great arcs.

The fog was hushed by the sound of the scythes moving through the fog. Soldiers

The fog was a constant reminder of their nervousness. Some were pacing and looking for disturbances, others were scanning the fog with an anxious eye. But none of them were too far from the field. Their throats were quiet except for a occasional grunt and groan. The reapers made quick, powerful sweeps through the field, and reached the middle of the field in no time. They stopped briefly to take a deep breath and wipe their sweat away before moving on towards the retreating sentry.

The sentry quickly moved towards the reapers and jerked his musket up.

slowly lowering his head and moving behind him. The eerie silence was broken by a spine-tingling cry. The sentry turned and fired, but then collapsed to hear a dozen flashes of light in the fog.

Stark eyes gazed down at the crumpled soldier, and immediately reacted.

Fear brought them to their knees. They ran to the tree, their arms reaching out in anticipation and grasping for air. Brady ran madly in front, trying unsuccessfully to outrun the painted devils rising above the fog. Spears landed on the ground and bobbed in his wake. The fog was stung by flashes. They all ignored him, except for the panting breaths that were coming from his heels. He did not look at the others and jumped to the ground to grab his rifle.

He cocked his weapon, rolled it over and fired it in one smooth shot.

Motion, falling his pursuer. Brady's bullet sent the painting brave reeling backwards. Blood spurted from his arm and his rifle flew into the wheat.

Brady spun, crawled frantically, and grabbed at the stubby.

He used wheat to help him get to the tree. He heard Thuds in the ground, wheat flying through the air from his grasp. He was not alone. More demons in the fog rushed towards him and began screaming, running away from them. He sat down on his knees and reached for the tree to grab one of the rifles. Then he turned around blindly to fire into a mass o' painted flesh at him.

There were many hands, shouting tongues, and angry feet that assaulted the victim.

He was a writhing man. He spun and tumbled among them. One strong hand lifted his neck and grabbed a handful of his red hairs. His hair fell from his head in a smooth, quick motion.

Other white men began to peel away and break in every direction. The fog greeted soldiers as they stumbled, only for them to hear a whizzing sound and see feathered spears flying close to their heads. They looked and fired into the fog, before rejoining their retreating comrades. The cursing corporal spotted them and ordered them to stop at the field's edge by the ridge. He began to count them and found two more missing, along with the unlucky sendry. He was only surrounded by four nervous people.

"Load! Damn you! He ordered, raising his arms.

Your musket to the field. The fog was shattered by yellow and red flashes. Each of the men followed him with his musket. He saw them disappear as his finger pressed the trigger. He was turned around by the sound of his men raising their weapons towards their shoulders. He moved the bayoneted musket's end towards the fog.

Brady groaned and twisted as he squirmed in the thick.

fog at the tree, just outside the sight of the corporals and his men. His body was ablaze from the stings and blows that he received. His scalp was burning, and blood was rushing into his eyes. He felt a small thud in his head, which made his eyes even more blind. He glared at the miscreant with a tomahawk, striking at his head in the direction of an older chief. He was a boy! A boy assaulted him now!

Brady stared disbelievingly at the brazen chief laughing at him

child's efforts. The chief ignored the look of the white demon and took the boy's hand. He raised the hand high and directed the boy on how to deliver a good blow.

The boy was able to take the lesson.

Brady was smashed by the tomahawk. Bright blue and black

His vision was flooded with thousands of tiny specks, which for a brief moment were blinding. He laughed and smirked at his adversaries. His sight was quickly covered in blackness. He gasped and fell into unconsciousness.

All soldiers stopped suddenly and turned around to face a comrade.

Rush to their side. They stopped abruptly, staring at the fog behind them as the four cradlers gasped. They also noticed the wide-eyed corporal.

One of them whispered, "What?" "You ain't thinking on," one of them said in a whisper.

You are going to die in the fog? You all will be killed if you do!"

The air rang out with a series of cries. The soldiers looked at each other.

Turned towards the cradlers and corporal.

"We should return to Wallis's, and spread the word!" One of the

The cradlers turned and ran up the hill, saying "Afford us all to lose our scalps!" "Before we all lose the scalps!"

One of the remaining cradlers stated, "He's right corporal." "The

You can't blame others for running away. You're only responsible for your hair falling out if you go into the fog. We're going to Wallis's, if we can do it!

The corporal gazed down at the fog. "It would most

He said, "Imprudent." "We will make our way back towards the fort by road until we meet a relief group."

The soldiers began to move back from the field and made their way home.

Through the thick fog, make your way to the road. They stood ready to face any demon that darted from the fog with their fury, their firelocks aimed at the surrounding fog. There was nothing that could be done to help the poor souls who were left behind in that field. Each one reasoned to himself.

A soldier who is dead did not do any good except the enemy.

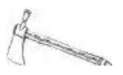

Chapter Eleven

He was able to roll along the grass. He rolled along the grass, his mind still numb. These visions were impossible to be true.

His eyes were forced open by a sudden, sharp pain. He was shocked. His scalp was charred. His arm was numb. His skin was swollen with cuts. Each pulse of blood to his brain made his brain throb. As he tried to open his eyes fully, dried blood stuck to his face. The dried blood around his face was covered in matted hair that grew from his fringes. It happened! His thoughts were filled with horror. His mother! His father! His brothers! Oh, my God! Never to see their faces again. Never again to breathe in the morning air, tinged by the morning dew. Never again to see the sunset. Never again to feel. He felt empty and cheated. He felt empty and robbed by the gift of life.

He still breathed and he saw the gritty with his face.

ground. He exhaled and dust flew from his face. He felt the dust settle on his head. But, strangely, he was open to the pain. To feel pain, one had to live.

He turned his head away from the dust. He raised his right.

But, it throbbed in opposition. He reached for his left hand and pulled it from underneath his body to wipe his eyes. Through the fog, he could see glimpses of the sun. It shone brightly with the promise of the next day. He survived! In terrible pain! He survived!

He sat still and listened, knowing that he wouldn't live long if he didn't.

None of the Indians saw him. To his immense relief, none the terrible devils of forest came near him. No one moved through the wheat stubble. They didn't let their tired, guttural voices drift through the air. They were gone! They had fled to hell and left their victim dead. But, wait! But wait! They must still be around! He gasped for air and yelled as loudly as his pain-filled lungs would allow. He didn't get a response. He must find them. At the very least, he must gain shelter in the cabin. Either the devils, or his comrades would return. He needed to be prepared for either.

He raised his hands to his scalp, and it was tingling with an awful sensation.

Burning pain. No! It's too fragile! You won't ever do it again. He slowly lowered his cursed fingers to his eyes and stared in amazement at the red liquid dripping from his hands. He felt a new gush of liquid from the area he had touched. He scolded him again, this time loudly. "No touching!" He noticed a brown substance sticking out of some matted wheat. His eyes lit up. His rifle! He had somehow escaped the attention of his torturers by grabbing it! He crawled to it and greedily grasped his arm to hold it. It felt good to feel the cold steel of the barrel. He wiped his eyes to get rid of any blood dripping into them and stared up at the ridge. It was just beyond the cabin!

> He stumbled to his feet and threw his rifle behind him, pulling it by the barrel.

He walked through the field. He struggled to get his feet over the field, fell once and quickly recovered his footing to continue his march to the cabin.

> He stumbled past wheat sheaths, some of which were smoldering from half.

They are attempting to set them ablaze with their hearts. "No, oh, no! He stumbled past the last tree on a ridge and mumbled, "Good Lord, don't let them have burned the cabin!" It brushed his face once more, falling against the rough bark. It stood, despite the last fogginess. It was the cabin! The chimney still has smoke!

> He yelled, "Halloo!" "Halloo! "Halloo!

For a long time, he waited for someone to come in the door. He shook his head and tried to make another sound before he collapsed to the ground from exhaustion.

"James!" A voice called from the shadows of the cabin door. "Is

that you?"

Brady gasped and lifted his head. "Old man!"

The elderly man stepped in front of the door, looking out carefully before

He ran to the tree, stumbling. He dropped the knife and poker he had in his hands and he lowered himself to the bleeding and suffering soul below with overwhelming pity.

He cried, "Oh, my dear God! It is you!" Brady Cradling's head in

He crossed his arms and gazed at the bloodshot and swollen eyes in front of him. He pulled out a rag from his pocket and wiped his face with it. He held it up to Brady's red, bleeding head. But he pulled it back as if he was going to make it worse by touching the wound. He asked, "Can you get up?" "It's best to get in the cabin."

He answered with a mournful groan.

Van Ness, an old man, lifted him by his arms and he fell to the ground.

Finally, he was able to get past the man-sized man. He led him to a bed and helped the poor soul to sleep on it. They were tough! He was there! He quickly tore his shirt into long strips and tried to bandage the wounds of the man in pain. He wiped more blood off Brady's face and sighed relief to see the blood stop flowing from his head. The thought of the pain inflicted on him made him wince. It must be very painful to have your hair taken out of your skull while you are still alive. He thought it was more painful than a ball. He quickly lifted a bandage to check Brady's right shoulder. It also stopped bleeding. It stopped bleeding at Brady's stomach. He smiled slightly. Even though he had only half-digested his stew, he recognized it immediately. He could not hide his horror when he looked at the spear wound. How is this man still alive? He thought to himself. He said, "You're going to need some stitchin', you are.".

"I will need more than that."

"Man, Brady's stuff is the heart of the earth.

are."

"You know what it is, old man. I don't want it any more."

soon."

Both men were nearly thrown to the ground by the sound of a turkey being eaten. What is a turkey? After all the chaos this morning, there would not be any. You could only be one thing. It could be a savage!

Brady called for his rifle, trying unsuccessfully to get out of the shackles.

bed. "My rifle! "Old man!" "Fetch my rifle!"

Unmistakable sound of a turkey's wings taking to flight

They were startled again for a heartbeat and a great feeling of relief. The old man replied, "T'was a Turkey after all, daggunit!" "Why will I be dipped into shit?"

Brady's fearful eyes glowed in his eyes. Recovering on the bed

He looked at the elderly man with deep concern. He said, "You need to get out of here." "They'll come back to finish their terrible work. There's no reason for us to be killed.

"Now, you must stop that foolish talk!

Old man said. "Ain't nobody leavin'' you in such an state!" He looked at the others and rolled his eyes as he thought of their hasty retreat.

Brady stared at Brady with his glassy eyes. He said, "I thirst." He said, "I thirst."

something terrible."
Van Ness looked around the cabin and finally found a small rum.

barrel. He said, "It's dried." "Damn fools drank all of it."

Brady's eyes were rolled left to right. He listened carefully.

The old man was looking at me again. He said, "The river." "Get me to that river!"

Van Ness assisted him with no protest and did not want to leave

He resisted his will. It proved to be a strong will, stronger than any he had ever known.

They found a few rods in the woods and headed down to the beach.

From the river to a landing in a canoe. Brady fell onto the sandy beach and sank his lips in the water. Brady gulped heavily for several minutes before he gasped, "my rifle old man, fetch your rifle!" He then immediately sank into the cool water, desperately trying to quench his thirst.

Soon, the old man appeared with a gun and Brady's.

rifle. He carried a cartridge case over his shoulder. Poor soul took the ball between his eyes and got it from one of the soldiers.

Brady raised his head from the water and stared blankly at the surface.

Old man. He stopped blinking hard, twice more, before he fell to the ground. Through his pain, he said "Load that old man!" "Load It!" He pulled his rifle pouch from his neck and raised it above his head.

Van Ness stated, "Now, be cautious." He advised that he take care of his wounds.

Brady's flailing arms were slowed down by his gingerly sliding the pouch with its powder horn under his shoulder and neck. Brady watched closely as he loaded the rifle. He said, "There," and closed the rifle's mouth by clicking its pan. It's all loaded up and primed.

Brady grabbed the weapon with his right arm and held it in his hands.

He felt like a newborn baby and fell to the ground. He immediately fell to the ground and fell into deep sleep.

The elderly man quietly loaded his gun, keeping his ears open for any possible danger.

His eyes were open for any movement and he made a lot of noise. He sat down beside his friend, wounded, after he had loaded. He stared up at the sky, thinking for a moment. "Lord! I know I haven't been very good at praying, but I'm calling upon you now. He said, as he looked down at Brady, who was in pain in his sleep and writhing in pain, "if not for my sake." Why should anyone die if they have such a will.

It is not a shame to be a shame. Amen."

He heard a rushing sound in his back. He stopped listening and froze.

He is being dragged closer by his creeping steps. He muttered, "This is it", and cocked his musket.

Brady was instantly awakened by the click. He jumped up and raised his arms.

He quickly raised his weapon and pushed the old man aside. He stared at the barrel of the rifle and glowed into incredulous eyes. He gasped and lowered his rifle to relieve himself. It fell on the ground in a lump. He gasped at his pain as he looked up at the men, their eyes fixed on him. My Ma! She is my Ma! I need to go to Sunbury.

Captain Walker kneels next to the victim and says, "Yes, definitely."

man. He looked at him in amazement as he continued to breathe God's sweet breath. He smiled at the old, teary-eyed man beside him and nodded. "Yes, absolutely, we can."

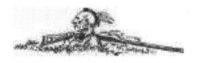

Chapter Twelve

Colonel Butler asked "Lieutenant Gore sir, what's all this about?" He was peering into the makeshift pine bough hut of the officer.

Slowly, the officer lifted a blanket and rolled on the hard ground.

He sat up and lifted his arms. He wiped his eyes and looked at the man in front of him. The other officers who shared the hut raised an irritated grunt. One of the officers smacked his lips and made a disgusting eye at the man. He was not affected by the man's cold stare. He rolled over and lifted his blanket above his head, grateful that he did not hear any protests from the stern-eyed officer.

Gore stretched and asked, "Colonel Butler?" He stood up groggily.

He was fumbling for his hat as the morning light dawns. "Assembly is not sounded, sir,"

Butler folded his arms and looked down at the row of huts, before taking a step back. "Are your sir, officer?

Gore replied, "Yes sir." Following his lead, he walked up to the colonel.

eyes. He noticed the mess in the men's huts immediately. He rubbed his forehead, then he let out a sigh. All hell would break loose.

Butler said, through his gritted teeth: "Orders" are that subaltern

Officers visit the guards during the day and inspect the soldiers' homes at night." He shoved his toe into a pile filled with noggins and trenchers that was piled up in front of the hut. He kicked at an iron pot and it clanged into another hut. He stooped over the hut, his hand resting on his waist. He pushed the blanket door open and reacted to the pungent scent. He gasped, "Huts and cooking tools must be kept clean, and clothing should be aired daily," he stated.

"Yes sir, but these men are too tired to finish these walls.

They're tired from scouting.

"You're a good officer with a commission.

sir?"

Gore did not say anything, but he just nodded his head.

"I'm sure Colonel Wisner maintained proper military bearing.

Butler stated that this was especially true when Butler spoke in front of the troops. Your fine service to him is proof that you are a good officer. Discipline is essential, even though we may be a little too independent. You know that men like ours are so resistant to resistance they must be led. Otherwise, they won't be driven."

Gore stated, "I know fair enough, Colonel, because I'm of the same stock.".
"Yes, I. It will be gone. It is the battlefield beyond.

The river is a testimony to the fact that popular rule has no place here. We must make sacrifices to survive. I promise you that we will survive." He gestured to the gate with his hand. The three settlers stood there looking tired from their long trek through the wilderness. The sentry stood nearby and he turned his cold gaze to him.

Gore recognized Abel Yarington as one of the men who had kept the journal.

ferry across the river. He raised his hand and waved at the sentry. The sentry was happy to resume his position. Gore felt an uneasy gaze on the nape of the neck and turned his attention to the stiff colonel in front of him.

Butler stared at Gore but nodded to Abel.

Yarington nodded, raising an eyebrow at Butler. War

He thought that men had brought out the devil in them. He rubbed his chin and moved towards the packhorses. He said, "Well, here are your things, Zebulon. On this horse." After he turned away, he led the three horses and two men off. Butler replied, "I am to look around my house, if not you mind.".
Grunting, Yarington lifted the rifle he had in his hands to his.

chest. "This is all I need for security, there's no need to fuss about it."

Butler shook his head and turned to Gore. "You have in your

He asked, "Could you charge three sergeants with five rank-and-file?".
"Yes sir."
"Gather this horse, and among other things on it, will you find a marquee.

Make some poles and erect them with great haste.

"Due haste?"
Butler replied, "Yes," and added that "you have your orders." It will be, I expect.

We will make use of it. It should be placed next to the great tree. It will be used for court martial. It will be of great benefit until discipline is restored, I fear.

Just to the opposite side of the room, a loud grunt from a hog was heard.

Stockade seemed to be answering the colonel. For a moment, he stopped to listen to the rutting beast. He rubbed his nose and said that the number of hogs in the area was too high. Since their owners were not there, it would be best to kill them for the soldiers. All such animals should be brought to the Commissary. They will need to be described and weighed. The Commissary will then pay the money at the usual price for the owner's use.

Gore replied, "Yes sir," and he looked to the untidy pine bough homes soon.

To be kept closed, it must be checked daily. This alone would likely fill the marquee in with many courts-martial.

Chapter Thirteen

Great huzzas roared down the mountains and rivers of Wyoming. In salute, the Cannon boomed along with the muskets. A column of Continental Line soldiers marched into the common, waving their hats in the air to relieved faces. The frowns of the column's gloomy faces were transformed into great smiles when the men in the column reached out to touch their backs. Their throats began to erupt with equally enthusiastic huzzas.

An officer in uniform with a red sash around his waist.

Horse to a stop infront of the column, and galloping to another officer standing before the fort.

The officer standing in front of the fort was clearly of high rank and stood beside his

His hands were cocked at his waist, his smile so big it threatened to burst. He extended his hand towards the officer.

Another round of huzzas was heard.

In salute, the mounted officer took off his hat.

Handing over a copy his orders to the officer in waiting; a colonel not less.

The colonel quickly stuffed the papers into his pocket.

He extended his hand once more. He said "No," and extended his hand again. Your presence is overwhelming!

The officer immediately smiled. Donning

He threw his hat on the colonel's head and accepted his welcome hand. "Captain George Bush," he said. He suddenly forgot the tiring march, his torn clothes and countless aches. "Captain Hartley's Regiment, awaiting your orders sir, with this fine detached of the same," he added.

All the men heard a thunderous roar. Both officers

The Captain Bush dismounted, and the Captain Bush eagerly shook hands with the other.

Bush graciously let go of his grip on the hand of the colonel

Straightening his clothes, he bows to all the congratulatory words and warm greetings.

"Fine sir. I am Colonel Butler commanding, Camp

"Westmoreland," the officer introduced him. He nodded his head and waved his hand towards his gate, leading the captain into the fort. He noticed the finely cut cloth that made up his uniform as he looked over at the captain.

He wore the shirt with pride even though it was a bit ragged and torn. It seemed to fit him perfectly. He seemed of good stock, and his manners and bearing seemed only to compliment his own style. Butler was afraid that he might have welcomed a dandy into the ranks.

Butler opened the cabin and asked, "What do I think of dance?"

door.

Captain Bush raised an eyebrow when he heard the strange question.

He was completely unprepared to answer such a question. He smiled and surveyed the posture of the colonel before he took the place at the table. He knew these were New England troops of puritan heritage and carefully chose his answer. He said, "I consider the art of dancing indispensable to the character a gentleman or an officer, sir," while watching Butler's sour expression overtake and destroy his smile. He added, "Just like His Excellency General Washington," for good measure.

Butler raised an eyebrow. Butler raised an eyebrow.

He said that the survival of the frontier and its necessities necessitates the exclusion from frivolous distractions such as dancing and playing cards. I am certain His Excellency would reach the same conclusion under such circumstances. For our very existence, it is essential to maintain discipline. Each man must rise above his faults and do his duty.

> Bush replied, "Yes sir," and he took off his hat. He sat straight in the chair.

As he did before his school marm in youth, he sat down on a chair.

> Butler stated, "I'm sure you saw the marquee under the tree green.".
>
> Bush nodded, vaguely recalling the water stained, torn.

A large, frayed tent was found partially patched. He mused, suddenly flushed with the thought that this was his headquarters.

> "I brought it here to hold the item."

Butler stated that it has courts-martial. It has been very busy of late. Your men are of a proper disposition, so I hope they don't agitate the situation at the moment.

> "No sir. I assure you that Colonel Hartley would not approve of it." We,

Sir, these are soldiers of The Line."

> Butler suddenly looked at the door and said "Yes," before he said it.

Closed properly. He marched over to the latch string and pulled it in. "Privacy is another reason that I called you within these wall, lest there be a marquee. All are open to hearing your thoughts. Some matters are best kept secret, as instructed by Colonel Hartley." He raised a piece of paper to the light from a single tallow candle. He has decided to march against the enemy at my request and that of others, as he sees the frontier's full extent impossible to defend with the forces at hand. Wyalusing was chosen by him as the point of departure for this expedition. I will inform you upon your arrival and send an express from Wallis's Fort Muncy. He has assembled a smart group of men around Wallis's. We will be moving upriver towards Tioga to meet Lieutenant Colonel Butler, Fourth Pennsylvania Regiment. We will then advance against Chemung, and wipe out all Indians and Tories from the river. It is quite ambitious, but it is necessary, I must admit. The matter will be most carefully considered. Secretariat is essential. "I am afraid Indian Butler and the Johnsons do not have ears around here yet," he said.

Captain Bush carefully read the text in the pale light. After

He read it and sat down on the table, rinsing his chin. He said, "My men are filthy." "I will have to inform Colonel Hartley about their most harrowing condition from their trek through wilderness to get to this place." He thought back to the similarly ragged appearance of the troops greeting him. "The men need new hunting shirts, and leggings in dire need."

Butler said "As is we all," pulling on his frazzled regimental.

coat. He regretted the action when he heard the seams being ripped. "But we all don't complain. The war is such, and our duty so serious it prohibits us from having such wants. However, I also wrote to the Council of War regarding the matter. I also hope that they will act quickly."

Bush said "Indeed", turning his gaze towards the door. The clamor

The cabin was awash with the excitement outside. "But I see that neither company lacks spirit."

Butler stated, "That is the most certain." "And if spirit are the true,

We have nothing to be afraid of in our arsenal of war. Its presence will make our enemies quake."

Bush smiled and accepted a mug full of rum.

Butler placed it in front of him. Both of them drank a lot from their mugs and slammed the plates down on the table. They both exclaimed, "Huzza to it!" and left the cabin to join the celebration.

Chapter Fourteen

Even though they had left Camp Westmoreland many hours ago, Isaac Tripp still remembers the cold stare of Colonel Butler. Tripp thought about the colonel's objections to him visiting his cabin on the Lackawanna River. In the past month, no one had been there. The river's upper reaches had not heard anything except for the terrible fate of St. John or Leech. Butler spoke of the importance and beauty of the crops, but did not know the extent of the destruction to the towns along the Lackawanna. He had protested to the colonel, who was a strong man, and he would have done so with his grandson, as well as two young militia volunteers. He was still beaming with gratitude for the two young men who offered to accompany them. They had finally put the colonel to his feet.

Un certain young man noticed his smile and smiled at him. "No

"No worries, Mr. Tripp," said he, rubbing his rifle's stock. "Powder, ball and all"

He laughed at the strange phrase repeated by Captain.

Bush's men, until Camp became a topic of conversation for everyone.

Westmoreland. Although most of Bush's men were Pennamites, they seemed to be a decent bunch. They didn't seem to care about Penn's claims against Connecticut settlers, but they were only concerned about their duty to the frontier. They knew that the more they could stop the Indian and Tory menace from their homes, then the better. They shared the same spirit, undoubtedly. American spirit.

Tripp and his friends raced past the cabins and burned mills as Tripp and his group ran.

Just above the remains of Pittston Fort. As they passed the carcass a single oxen, its rotting flesh prickling in spears and lances, Mrs. Leech's haunting words played on each of their imaginations. This is where St. John, Leech and their bodies were taken prisoner in the battle between three great power. They paid the price for their patriotism and simple honor. They looked at the two hurriedly made dirt mounds marking their graves on the road and were thankful that someone had the foresight to stop them.

They were all gone.

One particular cabin caught Tripp's attention, so much that he stopped before it. He was familiar with the cabin. He knew that the Hickmans had stopped at the cabin and refused to travel any further, knowing no harm would come to them this far upstream. He saw their bodies, including the infant son, woman, and man, in the ashes. His mouth opened with an anguished gasp.

His grandson, who stopped and stared at the sky, asked "What's it Papa?"

He stood in the charred cabin and wondered what horrors he had seen through his grandfather's eyes.

He said, "The Hickmans." "You still remember them?"

"Yes, Grandpa, I do."

"Well, that's all they have left."

His gaze was pierced by a call from the top of the trail. Two militiamen arrived.

They waved them up to the trail, at the crest of the ridge.

The old man nodded. He lowered his gaze to the cabin and then he put his hand on his.

He placed his hand on the shoulder of his grandson. He said that he would return and ensure his grandson received a proper burial.

The men exhorted them to "Come, Come", appearing excited by the opportunity.

They can see something below them. They anxiously fidgeted nervously with their rifles, lifting them to their shoulders and then slowly lowering them.

Old Tripp squirmed, looking down at the gap below. It's only Leggett's Creek.

"Jim could have sworn he saw one among 'em darting away into them

Trees by the creek!" One of them replied.

Tripps searched the gap below intently for signs.

Movement. Their anxious minds were eased by the sight of a turkey walking along the bank.

Tripp, the elder, asked: "Are these the feathers that you saw young Hocksey?"

asked.

Jim almost laughed in relief, and he shook his head. The other raised his eyebrows.

Take aim at the turkey with your rifle.

"No! No! Timothy," Tripp, an old man, said. Tripp said, "If there aren't any Injuns around that shot will certainly bring them about!"

The young man quickly lowered his rifle and was stunned.

embarrassed.

Tripp stated, "It's all good." Tripp said, "No harm done."

His shoulder. "We are about twenty miles from the nearest post. It is important to keep an eye on everything. You'll be fine. Just lay low."

Timothy Keyes stated, "My land is just a few kilometers ahead."

He lifted his head again, and regained his composure. Everyone saw the new sparkle in his eyes. He was the Pittston Company Ensign, and his military mentality took control of his demeanor. "We'll stop here and then push on towards Hocksey's, then yours, Mr. Tripp."

Both Hockseys and Tripps nodded. Slowly, they made their way to each other.

Each one of them looked more closely at the trees and shrubs as they made their way down the trail towards the creek. Keyes glanced at the creek and tried to find rocks to cross the creek. He ignored the tingling sensation at his neck. When they sprung onto him, he just put his foot on the rock. They were surrounded by dozens of painted men, each one staring at them deathly.

Nobody spoke. The white men watched as the scene unfolded and froze in place.

The Indians were circling. Some brave men pointed rifles at them from within a few feet of each other's faces. Others held tomahawks or spears in threatening poses. The Indians looked at the white men and almost dared them to raise their rifles. However, something in their dark eyes warned them what would happen to any white man who even moved a muscle.

Finally, one of the faces was painted and a wild scream broke out.

The sheer force of the impact caused the warrior's head and neck to sway backwards. The sharp sound of the turkey's wings made a loud thud. Squirrels ran madly up the trees. The shivering wail caused birds to take flight. The forest was seized by the apex predator.

Tripp, an elderly man, let go of his grip and let his rifle fall helplessly.

The ground. He looked at the screaming warrior and motioned slowly for his grandson. He also saw his grandson drop his rifle to the ground.

Hocksey looked in terror, wide-eyed Each warrior was instantly able to respond.

He started screaming, the forest echoing his taunts. His rifle fell from his shaking hands involuntarily.

Keyes stood still in mid-stride above the rushing waters. He was a good man.

All of them would be sent to Hell or Tioga if they were fired, but the worst outcome seemed insignificant. The touch of his finger on a trigger could save lives. One shot is better than at least twelve. He was gripped by fear and mutely muttering prayers amid the screaming demons.

He was accompanied by a huge warrior who jumped into the stream next to him. Raising his

Tomahawk high above the stunned Yankee, he brought it down beside Keyes, only slicing at his air to warn him. He clenched his teeth and thumped his large chest in the most grizzly way, leaving indentations in paint.

Keyes sat in stunned silence as he watched. He wanted to move.

His rifle was ready to be used against the demon. But his muscles became stiff. The warrior stood still as he reached for his rifle, touching it gingerly.

The warrior, sensing no resistance, jerked the weapon away.

He splashed back at the others. He raised the weapon high above his head in triumph and screamed at his highest lungs. Keyes was knocked to the bottom by two warriors. After a few fights, Keyes was finally pushed to the bottom by two warriors. He was thrown to the banks of the creek by a massive warrior in one motion.

In an attempt to keep the hands of young Yankee men in touch, leather thongs were used.

instant. They were draped with looped hemp ropes. The warriors showed their teeth and yelled at Tripp to make them submit before his shocked eyes. He stared through his tear-strewn eyes in horror as he stood still.

A similarly old warrior stood next to the tree, rising from the forest.

The old white man. He crossed his arms and stood steady between the older man and the younger soldiers.

Both were ignored by the warriors, who continued to search for their own treasures.

Through the young captives' bags and haversacks. The older warrior tilted his head and looked out from the corner of his eyes at his elder brother. He reached into his pocket and waved a hand at one of the young gallivanting braves. He reached into his pouch and pulled out a small pot of clay. He eagerly rubbed the clay with his fingers. He turned towards the white man and smeared the vermillion paint all over his face.

He waved his hand along the trail, "Jogo!" "Jogo!"

Tripp, an old man, stood stunned for a second and cursed himself.

Insistence on the expedition being undertaken in the first instance. Colonel Butler didn't seem so foolish now. He opened his mouth and looked among the young men trying to keep a calm but sincere eye on his grandson. He was sent reeling backwards by a gruff push to his chest, which sent a torrent of tears down his cheeks.

"Jogo!" The old warrior yelled again, this time using a cutting motion.

His neck. His eyes bulged. He turned his attention to the yelling soldiers and the stunned white man who was falling to the ground beneath his shaking feet. He said "Jogo!" again, scratching his skull, "You die too, if there is no jogo!" He raised his arms in frustration.

The white old man tried unsuccessfully to turn his back, but stumbled to his feet.

He turned his head away from the scene in front of him. He uttered words of a prayer that he didn't know but would accept. He finally turned his eyes away from his grandson, and began to walk madly down the trail. Feeling so deeply remorsed, his vision was clouded by the tears. He wept openly as he fell just above the crest of the ridge. He could hear the screams of the warriors echoing through his head from one ear and another. He cried out, "Why?"

His plea was answered by another terrible scream. His wide eyes darted

back towards it. He continued to walk down the trail, his heavy feet allowing him to hear the horrible sounds. He stumbled and grabbed any branch or tree he could to escape the haunting vision of death that was haunting him.

He sobbed, "Oh dear Lord!" "Hell has returned to Wyoming!"

Chapter Fifteen

Young Isaac Tripp saw his grandfather's back fall over the top of a crest. A hollow feeling filled his heart. He realized that he had never felt so alone before. He was alone and had lost all dignity and integrity in one fell swoop. He closed his eyes and felt a single tear run down his crimson cheek. His eyes were forced open by a slap.

Hocksey stood barely in front of one of the demons.

His knees were shaking. He was surrounded by a heathen, who bowed down to him in all his glory, his eyes glistening with the power of death or life. The demon painted in full spit on the young, white man's face and gruffly shoved him to the ground.

Hocksey looked pleadingly at Tripp as he rolled over.

Tripp shook his head. His quivering lips did not respond to the words he was uttering.

Keyes demanded, through the yells, "Leave Him Be!".
Each shaking shook the warriors as they looked at him in contempt.

They turned their heads at the young man. One of them pulled his knife out of its sheath, and placed it in his mouth. He mockingly acted like he had cut his tongue with it. With a sparkling eye, he nodded at the young white man.

Keyes took the hint. He bowed in silence. He was a rough yank

The rope wrapped around his neck made it difficult for him to raise his head again. He felt a burning sensation as the rope tightened around his neck.

He said nothing, despite the pain. His Adam's apple rose, and fell.

He clenched his throat and tried to stop his fearful cry. They wanted it. They wouldn't get it from him.

The old warrior entered the melee and raised his hands.

He cursed at the bravest. He shook his head and pointed at the creek. He yelled, "Jogo!" "Jogo!"

After a few half-hearted protests from the warriors, they took up the challenge.

Tethers were tied around the necks of their captives. They raced straight up the bank to the opposite bank and did not wait for their bound captives' balance to be re-established. They pulled them along, pulling at the tethers mercilessly.

They were quickly scolded by the old warrior who brought up their rear.

Their native tongue. One of them retaliated, but everyone stopped. The captives were able to regain their feet on the leaf-strewn bank. After a brief pause, they walked along the edge of the gully on a narrow trail with branches snapping into their faces. They closed their eyes and waited for the next blow, not having any hands to stop the limbs from piercing their faces. They endured the pain silently and praised God when the branches stopped stinging them.

They all poured after hurriedly passing through Leggett's Gap.

Out onto a clearing on a small plateau. The lead warrior moved slowly to the edge of the clearing and motioned for the other soldiers to stop. This relief was felt by the young white men. All of them gasped for air as they struggled against the tight ties around their necks.

The giant warrior at the front stood tall and surveyed the surroundings.

The clearing. His hard eyes remained fixed on the beleaguered and gasping prisoners. He rolled his eyes away from them and called for his fellow soldiers to gather around him. After a while, they spoke for a while, looking back at each other and laughing occasionally, before suddenly stopping.

The old warrior, seemingly not invited, stood aside to the side the

Clearing his throat, he mumbled to himself and moved to and fro. His throat was full of loud complaints, but he could not suppress them. His rantings were ignored by the younger warriors.

All of them rose slowly, circling the grieving boys without

They did not say a word. Then another one came to the boys and ran the hair of the boys through their fingers.

Young Tripp stood still, strangely realizing that his hat was still.

He wore it on his head. While the braves checked Keyes and Hockseys locks, he looked up at it. They quickly walked over to him, grabbed his locks, and then snatched the hat off his head.

Infuriated, the old warrior pushed into them, appearing furious.

They walked away from the terrified boy. He waved his arms towards the two other captives and took Tripp by the arm, leading Tripp over to the clearing's edge. He gently lifted the boy's hair and waved his other hand, cursing the soldiers. He removed the boy's hat and began to play with the one feather in his hair. One tear cut through his red and black cheeks, revealing the faint traces of a faded tattoo. He waved again at the white boys below and the gully. He reached for the small medicine pouch that was hanging around his neck and raised it to the heavens, asking for help from an unknown power.

It worked especially well when distant thunder clapped.

Boomed, appearing to answer the old man's prayers. The bulging eyes of the warriors stared upward at the heavens. The giant warrior shrugged his shoulders and pointed to the braver. The brave raised his spear in anger, but soon stopped under the threatening eyes of his companion.

He laughed and walked over to Tripp. He squats in front

He pulled Tripp by the neck lead and turned his back to his friends, leading Keyes & Hocksey into the gully. Tripp's deep concern was evident in his eyes as he pulled the lead from his neck until the Yankee's eyes were fixed on his.

Tripp stared at the breech-clothed with all his color loss

He was a warrior in front of him. The gruff brave had dozens of tattoos covering his entire body. One of them was a long snake tattoo that covered his entire forehead. A long line of triangles ran along his upper arms and torso, protruding all the way from underneath. Nearly every spot on his skin was covered by dots and small circles. Under his smiling mouth, a silver nosepiece was dangling. It exposed yellow-tinted teeth from smoking. Many smaller brass and silver ornaments were hung around the large cartilage loops that extended from his ears. Each of his arms was adorned with silver arm bands that hung around his biceps. His crown of hair sparkled with bear fat grease and had a single, erect feather stuck in it. Tripp couldn't have imagined how horrid he looked in front of Tripp. His breath was strange and bland, yet somehow sweetened by the scent of the herbs in the forest. The bulging white pits in his eyes, the dark hair on his head and no eyebrows. His hair was painstakingly trimmed to provide a better base for the paint that covered his body. He was a skilled warrior who had thousands of years of experience to see terror in the hearts of his adversaries. Now he was face-to-face with Tripp. The warrior's eyes showed the depth of the battle they fought. Tripp might be right, but those eyes did not show the slightest hint of mercy.

Both are recognized here, just a few breaths apart.

The vast and incalculable gap was created by a thousand life experiences of their own and their ancestors. These experiences were forged by two completely different cultures and lands. It seemed impossible to bridge the gap with just a few more generations. Both of them were shocked at the realization. This war, this clash between cultures, was not possible to avoid. It is true, but it is sad.

The old man grunted and both of their eyes were shattered. The old man walked slowly to the gully while watching the white boy, a warrior sitting in front of him. He cocked his head and crammed his hand against his ear, looking ahead. He shook his head in horror for a moment, but then his eyes grew tired and disappeared under his tired eyelids. He jerked his head and slowly moved back and forth before finally returning to the clearing. He folded his legs and sat down beside them. Tripp stared at him with apologetic eyes. He couldn't find words to express the pain in his eyes or heart.

From the gully below, the braves poured into the clearing. They laughed and nodded at each other, imitating their victims without much regard for Tripp or the old Indian.

Tripp felt his stomach turn sour. Tripp grins wide across the room

The brave face squats in front of him. The brave stood up and gestured for the prizes. He gasped and held the trophies that his fellows had given him high up, looking at them with a certain sparkle in his eyes. He was full of pride and walked over to Tripp to show the scalps. He first held the blond hair under his nose and twisted it before moving to the red. The hair was still tied with a ribbon. Tripp, a young man, had seen his hair bob up and back on the trail all day. His jaw dropped and his jaw relaxed.

Tripp was greeted by a huge warrior who marched up to him, and he slapped his hat.

His head. He grabbed his hair and pulled it taut at its roots.

The young, scared white boy let a tear slide down his face. He lowered his eyes and watched the warrior's hands drop to his belt. He closed his eyes and prepared for a hit from a tomahawk. He felt a rapid movement of air around his cheek and stood tall despite it. He thought, "Do your worst," You will not find the satisfaction of your fear. If my eyes betray, I will close them and bring them to Providence. He took a deep, exhaling breath, knowing it would be his last. His cheek felt tingly from the touch of a slap. He felt a wet sensation. He felt a pull at his wrists from the leather thongs. His hands were freed from the leather thongs and he felt his hands fall to his side.

He touched his face instinctively, feeling the wet sensation.

cheek. He stared at the red substance with awe as he extended his hands to his face. It was sticky, but not thick enough to be blood. It was thick and sticky, he sniffed it nervously to the laughter of the warriors. He realized that it was just paint!

In one smooth motion, the old man rose to his feet. You are now overpowered

He touched the paint on the boy's cheeks with relief. He started to laugh, but it was in a more innocent way. He said in English, "You live!" He added, nodding his head vigorously. "You live!" He pointed with his long, bony finger at Tripp, then pointed up towards the sky. "Hawenneegar!

Amazing spirit! You have his support today!"

Tripp looked in disbelief, then took a deep breathe and enjoyed it. Life,

Even as a captive, he never felt so happy. He applied the life-giving paint to his face with his fingers. He looked around in wonder and let out a giggle at the sight of his friend's hair tied around the waists of his captors. He wondered who had suffered the worst fate.

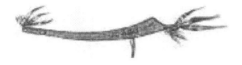

Chapter Sixteen

Tripp, an elderly man, sat in a large elm tree by the river common, his head down to his chest as he cried. His shirt was stained with red paint and dripped of tears. He repeated the words he said when he first appeared before the fort: "They've taken their!" Leggett's Creek! They've taken them!"

His grandson Giles Slocum took over immediately.

John Jenkins left with a rescue team to Leggett Creek, and John Jenkins was still there at his side the whole night. He tried to comfort him by listening to his grand-father's murmurs, even though doubt was tinged in his words. He stood firm, even through the most difficult day, and now he was watching as the sun sets with him.

Giles handed him a canteen with rum and said "Here Grandpa."

Take a piece of bread and "take this, you'll be well." Jenkins will bring you food, so you must eat. You'll need strength to get through the next round.

He said it all with his tired eyes, looking up at him. The old man was polite

Refused to eat the bread and instead drank a glass of water.

Slocum stated, "Well, at the very least, you're feeding yourself," eating.

The bread was made by him. He leaned against the tree, looking at the fire pit between the fort and tree, and nodded to the men who were standing with their arms folded, gazing at him. He was shaken by the two men who looked at him.

Nathan Denison stated, "He's taking this hard.".
Colonel Butler stated, "Yes, poor soul, indeed." What about what's?

These are difficult times for Luke Swetland, Blanchard. They're either in Tioga or Hell, but who knows? I personally pray for them both and Keyes, Hocksey and young Tripp to find heaven. I am afraid of the tortures these poor souls may have to go through."

Both men turned to music in the grim for inspiration.

The mood at the time. The pair stared at the silhouette of a man against the wall of Fort, following his precise movements to the rhythm of the lively music.

Denison stated, "I fear Captain Bush may be a little too dandy."
"Southern

People are a weird lot.

Butler raised his hand to his face and said "Yes, they're," "But

They are his musicians, and it seems that they have their own way."

"Nonsense especially in these times and in such places,"

Denison said that he was looking at a group women who had returned to Wyoming. Their stout, hardy frontier women seemed to share his dislike of young dandy acts. They watched in fascination as one of them nearly danced, while the other stared at the strange sight with cold eyes.

Butler: "It seems that Mrs. York wants join good Captain Bush."

said.

It is hard to imagine a New England woman joining the ranks of the

Denison let out a small laugh at the dignified captain. It was quickly put out by Denison when he saw the sad woman sitting next to Mrs. York. Yesterday's death of Mrs. Durkee's son was a heavy blow to her face. He thought of his son, who was the same age, and thought of his nosebleed. Hooker Smith's efforts as well as many others failed to stop the blood flow and the boy died in front of everyone. It was a tragedy, as he was the oldest son of Captain of First Westmoreland Independent Company, one of Wyoming's companies that fell on the battlefield of the last battle defending their homes.

He recalled that day vividly and the image of Mrs. York, a stubborn woman, begging to be released from the fort before it surrendered flashed through him again. Parshall Terry, the man who had taken her husband and made them homeless had demanded that she surrender. Parshall Terry, the rascal she called him, demanded her surrender. She was determined to kill the entire family in the fort. She was wrong but time proved her right. However, such feelings are just as painful as his stare at her now. He looked away, but she was still looking at him as he walked around the fire. To vent his frustration, he raised a hand.

Lucrietia York screamed, "Oh, my dear Colonels," as she positioned herself.

They will see you standing up for your cause. She brushed her hair back and turned her head toward them. She said, "No doubt that rascal Terry's about this mischief!".

Denison stated, "My dear Mrs. York, it is good to meet you." Butler

He just looked at her with his eyes closed and didn't say a word.

"My Amos was killed in Connecticut. I was heartbroken and thought we would never see him again."

She said, "All of them had been killed in that massacre." She looked up at the flames, her eyes glistening with tears. "No doubt from his, Fitch, and Jenkins' cruel imprisonments in that hellish hole of Fort Niagara. Fitch also passed, you know, shortly after his exchange." She shook her head and stared at Colonel Butler. "But, sir, you have chosen the right man to handle this matter about Leggett's Creek. Damn 'em, John Jenkins will cross paths with Terry the rascal or any of them. He'll only bring back the scalps of the thieving rascals. He's the man for this job!

Butler stated, "Well, I am glad some approve my decisions."

"Mrs. Terry is a lower lieutenant in their ranks than York.

Denison stated, "Give him too much credit.".

"Ya think?" Mrs. York asked. "Well, I tell you, and all of my

Children will too, because there is no greater devil in these parts than man or savage. You can be sure that if you get Tom Green and Thomas Hill the Tory dog, all this mischief will stop! That bit of wisdom is mine!

Butler stated, "We will deal avec traitors. I assure you.".

Lucrietia York looked with a smile towards Butler. "I

Fine sir, durst you say ye will. "I durst say that ye will," she said, and then turned to go back to the fire to be with Mrs. Durkee.

Butler stated, "That woman doesn't lack spirit."
Butler stated, "No," Denison replied, "but spirit does not equal everything.".
The other side of the president's marquee: A call from the other

Both of them were shocked. They looked at the men sitting next to it and saw Old Tripp suddenly rise up to his feet and take a few steps towards the road.

Denison asked, "Could it possibly be?".
Butler stated, "We can only hope," joining others who are expressing their dismay.

The fort to welcome a party marching down the street.

Wyoming's eyes were on the exhausted party as they trudged down the stairs.

Road towards them. The musicians of Captain Bush stopped playing. A few people cried out to the party only to hear a few muffled grunts echo back to them. Although Old Isaac Tripp was more stricken by the party's glum mood, it did little to dampen their spirits. He fell towards Lieutenant Jenkins, who looked crestfallen and shook his head.

The elderly man gripped him by the shoulders and stared in pain.

down to mother earth.
He gasped. He sucked hard, despite his overwhelming.

He was in grief and looked up at the lieutenant.

Jenkins said "No," and stepped off to the side. Bowing

He waited with his head for the colonels to come within earshot. He said, "We found nothing but two hats with a ribbon." "The hats belonged to Keyes, Hocksey. There was no sign of young Isaac. This is good, it means they've adopted them." He stared at the eyes of the elderly man. It's fine. He'll be fine. I should have known. I can assure you that they will treat him well. He'll be back after this horrible war is over.

Tripp wiped his eyes and said "Yes, young Jenkins", wiping away his tears. Tripp wiped his tears and said, "Yes, young Jenkins."

Let me know if you would. "I'll take your word for it."

Jenkins stated, "You have it." Jenkins said, "I only wish I could have caught you up."

"I was with them, and I relieved them of their charges and their scalps." He threw up in frustration. "But we did everything we could."

Tripp stated, "That's what you have," and "I, as well as all the others."

appreciate it."
Jenkins nodded and turned his attention to the colonels. Jenkins nodded.

They looked at him and let the man with the men stumble to the fort.

Denison: "Things are getting hotter in more than one way."

He wiped the sweat from his forehead.

Butler replied, "I know." "But Hartley is of the same mind as I. Protecting the frontier means striking at them in their homes. They are convinced that they can strike with impunity upon us, and so they sit around Tioga or Chemung. They must be convinced otherwise.

Denison stated, "That is what we must." "That is what we must."

Chapter Seventeen

The trees around Fort Muncy were haunted by a mist that rose in the early morning light. The men slowly awoke from their sleep to prepare for the new day. The fires blazed to life. Oxen and horses neighed. All the creatures of burden were silent except for the sentries who sat around the fort's half-finished walls. They seemed so calm and peaceful that they didn't pay much attention to the three men walking out the gate into the misty early morning.

One of them, who was afraid of the corporal of guard, was called back

They said in German, "Halt!" They turned and muttered something to the man before he waved off their protest.

Nothing was stirred between the stillness of the dawn, and the wild potatoes

The fort's location offered an appealing alternative to the bland meals. They worry too much, so they spoke in German together before continuing their journey. They walked three more steps before they stopped.

One pointed at the scrub brush right in front of him.

They stare at him, and he curiously tilts his head. A dozen rifles immediately began to chirp in the misty early morning. To the horror of his unarmed companions, the man stood straight up and gasped before falling to the ground. From the mist, yells were heard.

> "Mien Goot! "Das wildens!" one of the screamed, dropping his weapon.

bundle. He left his friend alone, and he turned to run pell-mell to the fort.

> A bold, white man dressed in a green jacket emerged from the mist to be seen.

He was accompanied by several painted men who emerged from the bushes behind him wearing a leather cap. The white man ignored the German in his path and knelt down to level his rifle against the back of the man running behind him. The man fired and a small amount of dirt flew between his legs.

> "Alarm! "Alarm!" was heard from within the fort. Drum

Assembly was defeated immediately. Numerous sentries were fired upon the men who emerged from the fog. In the fort, groggy voices yelled out urgent orders.

> "Damn!" The green-coated white man quickly replied, reloading his weapon.

He raised his rifle and looked at the rebel German militiaman in front of him, seemingly shocked.

> The German shouted "Tory dog!" and threw down his bundle. He he

Instantaneously, he rushed towards the green-coated miscreant with his eyes bulging from anger. The Indian stopped him from moving and aimed his tomahawk at the mad German.

The Indian was grabbed by the mad German and the German twisted the weapon.

He released his grip and sent him tumbling down to the ground. He became more furious when he saw the Indians mingling around his dead comrade's body. One of the men lifted his friend's bloodied scalp in the air. He lowered his head in an agonizing grunt and moved steadily towards them, seemingly unaware of their presence.

Tory said, carefully aiming his rifle. "He's a right smart man."

At him. He was tackling him from behind, but his target fell to the floor before he pulled the trigger.

The Tory raised his rifle and viewed the battle before him with an awe.

certain glee. His gaze was quickly broken by several whizzes around his ears. He pointed at one of the approaching sentries and fired. The ball thudded into the stockade behind him sending splinters flying through the air, as he watched. Slowly he backed into the scrub brush and shielding mist, shouting along with his Indian friends at the top of their lungs.

The Indian and the militiaman rolled around on the ground grunting.

groaning. Their hands were tightly wrapped around one another, as if they were grasping at the throats of their fellow man. Each of their fingers dripped blood, piercing each other's flesh. Both of them stumbled to their feet, refusing to let go of their death grips, shooting in the air. They could hear the dirt flying around their feet. The German grabbed the Indian and threw him in the brush with a single strong effort. The branches cracked and there was a loud groan in the air. The air was filled with the sound of feet frantically scampering through the brush in a flash.

The German fell to his knees and stared at his blank eyes, staring at the sky.

fallen friend. He grabbed large quantities of earth with his fists and flung them into the brush. He ignored the soldiers rushing around him and fired into the forest. He was overcome with grief and leaned over the body of his friend, weeping openly.

Colonel Hartley made his way through the field towards the

He waved for the men to hurry ahead of him, while holding a pistol in his other hand and clenching the blanket around him with the third. The grieving man stopped him from coughing and he hacked.

He turned his face towards the colonel in pain. He said, "Mien God Herr Colonel, mien God! Look at what das wildens did to poor Hans!" "I knew him well, and he was mien friend. Poor soul!" He began to pound his fists into earth with great thumps. "All we wanted was the bit of potatoes. That's it. These wildens must be stopped!

He bowed his head and cursed his feverish body. He turned

They heard the sound of hooves racing towards them. Captain Carberry crashed his horsesmen into the forest and yelled at the enemies.

Hartley said, shaking his head, "Too late.".

"Sir. A Tory was with them for sure, all dressed up in green he belonged."

Hartley was notified by an exasperated corporal, who looked down at Hartley and the fort just two rods from him. He rushed to reload his musket and saw Captain Walker emerge from the brush.

Walker stated, "No sign of them," and he doff his hat at Hartley.

"They've disappeared."
Hartley stated, "Yes," Hartley added, "something must now be done."

He moved one of his moccasins to the surface against the frosty ground. It crunched. Some trees showed a hint of orange and crimson. He wailed, "The season has got late and there is not sign of the Indians or Tories letting it up," he stated, wiping his nose in frustration. "Curse this damn fever! Without it, we should have been off against them weeks back!"

Walker stated, "The rains will start soon, sir.".
Hartley turned his cold gaze towards Hartley. Hartley said, "Give this poor soul a

Proper burial is required. I will send a dispatch to Bush, Hunter, and Butler. We will strike soon! We will strike soon!

"Yes sir," Walker said.
Hartley looked down at the bereaved German and said: "But keep it underneath your hat," Hartley said, gazing down at the grieving German, "No one is to speak a word!"

The German sorrowful soul stood, sobbing.

Walker said, "No worries sir," and took the man by his shoulder.

He was a guide to the fort. "I don't believe he's heard anything through his grief. Hartley was told by he that he would get the men ready under some pretense.

Hartley stared into the forest and said, "I hope so." "I do fear

These devils may only be defeated by our ability to surprise ourselves.

Chapter Eighteen

Robert Covenhoven moved with all of the grace and stealth that he had. He made a pacing over rocks, knowing that it would not leave any sign of his death. He knew the forest's eyes. Before all this trouble, he had traded with them and scouted. He was familiar with the trails, the red and white men as well as the enemies he encountered. He wondered if that is why William Stewart, his fellow scout, trusted him to go to Wyoming with the dispatches sewn into his hunting shirts. He felt the full weight of his mission as he thought about the fake dispatches in his pocket. The enemy would not suspect the real dispatches if he was captured.

Hartley believed in Hartley, and he was not without limits.

He would have faith in himself and his scalp.

He walked along the trail's edge, ready to leap behind a tree

At the sight of any one. He was not the only one who saw a patriot in his uniform. Yet, loneliness lingered in his heart. His heart sank against his chest with each rustle of deer or caw of a bird. In tight spots, two rifles were more effective than one. Hartley insisted on strict secrecy and whisked Stewart away in the middle of the night, with dispatches to his commanders. Hartley sent an officer to Stewart at the last minute, increasing his chances of making it. It all felt strange and he felt like he was being cheated. But duty called, and if he didn't answer, a second officer would be sent with Stewart.

He was frozen by a slight movement of red in his trees ahead

He stopped dead in his tracks. His eyes remained fixed on the movement. He carefully moved his body around the huge tree listening. Some song birds sang in the still air. A slight rush from the stream below mixed with the sounds - all normal sounds, no alarm sounds from man or beast.

He walked through the forest floor's great ferns, stumbling along.

He was careful not to disturb its animals, as he knew that his enemy depended on their warning. A few rustling sounds and distinctive guttural words were heard ahead. He listened to them and tried to understand the meaning of the conversation but the distance obscured it.

He needed to get closer. He slowly eased his rifle under the ferns, lowering himself to the soft soil. He moved his hand forward, then a leg back, and his eyes scanned the surroundings as he did so. His neck tingled. His senses were all unified. He shifted his attention towards a large, moss-covered rock above his prey and he continued to move in that direction.

The voices grew to be between two and three and finally to four. He finally stopped.

Just before the rock, I listened and considered making a detour along the trail. This was the end of the trail, which narrowed down to a steep gorge that was too steep for him to avoid. This was the only way he could go. He crept up to the rock's back, and he leaned his back against the soft moss. He waited for the enemy to move before nightfall, raising his rifle high up to his chest.

With each beat of his heart, moments ticked away. He sat in silence.

Move a muscle and listen intently to what is below. A fire crackled. He was relieved to hear his feet shuffle occasionally, but they remained away from him. He listened to their voices, one bragging, and another shaming everything the braggart said. One laughed, while another suggested that they follow the trail to attack the white-eyes as they sat in the forts. He pleaded for more scalps to Tioga. To see the Indians' land forever, more white-eyes were needed.

The argument finally grew in the natural world. The argument grew louder in nature.

Protest, only to be rebuked. These boasts were heard by even the white-eyes. To be one with the forest, one must lower one's voice and speak in harmony with it.

Covenhoven listened to his fears, afraid that if he retreats he would be

detected. He reached for his pistol in his sash, and his tomahawk. One shot, rifle, one gone. One shot, pistol. Two gone. Three shots, one throw of the tomahawk. But that left one. He was just as strong as the other. He was just as strong as the other. He flattened himself against the moss and silently prayed.

As the distance increased, one after another, the voices became fainter until they disappeared altogether.

Finally, only one remained and taunted the others as they fled. The sound of a faint rustle through the trees echoed over the moss-strewn rocks after the retreating taunts had ended. There were no voices in the air.

He lowered his head slowly towards the rock's edge. He was alone.

He was not far from his hideout when he turned back. The dying fire emitted smoke to the side. He watched as the muscles of his tawny back flexed and the hands worked hard on something. He couldn't see the problem, but prayed that it would be solved soon so they could both be on their way. Both his way and the other's, the latter not knowing that they had passed. He preferred this way of doing things. An alarm would sound if a rifle shot was made. We don't know how far his companions traveled up the trail?

He sat and watched as the back work was done. He felt his muscles rise and fall. The grunt of

Some exaggerated movements were accompanied by frustration. One hand raised a knife to the ground, while another raised a small sapling in his front.

He noticed the rifle of the brave lying on the ground to his right.

His pouch and tomahawk. The brave had very few other possessions. He must travel light or be part a larger war party near him.

He lowered his rifle to his chest and watched the trail go by.

right. He thought he could get past preoccupied brave if his pace was slow and he would be on the right side. The day grew longer. He couldn't waste any more time and had to get up quickly.

There was a gasp followed by a quick grunt and then a cheer.

Triumph, rise from the brave. The Indian raised his arms and gazed with pride at the trophy.

Covenhoven's jaw dropped. Covenhoven's jaw dropped from the weight of his long, flowing hair.

A sapling hoop is displayed in front of the brave. The hair of a helpless girl. His rifle was able to slide over the rock.

The brave senile moved in Covenhoven's direction suddenly sensing something. His whites were shining against the pale dusk light, his eyes sparkling brightly. Surprised, his eyes sparkle.

His eyes lit up in a flash. All his courage was lost when the brave fell.

He was deprived of all life except for the slight twitching in his hand, still holding the prize on the hoops.

Covenhoven ran past the rock from behind, darting out of the rock.

Indian twitching. He ran, his heart racing with the satisfaction of taking revenge on some poor woman and his fear for his life. No doubt, the others heard the shot. They would eventually find the body. The hunt might just be beginning.

Chapter Nineteen

Abel Yarington sat with his arms crossed across his chest, staring indignantly at those seated around his table. He gripped his slouchy hat tight in his hands and his fingers tightened. He tightened his grip, craning his hat into an ugly shape as he thought more about the court-martial's invasion of his home.

He worked tirelessly to repair his home, which was charred.

Standing picket duty, and other duties imposed by Colonel Butler on the local population Butler! He sat at the top of the table, shuffling papers and looking like a regal lord. The Quartering Act had the colonel never heard of it? This was the revolution! It was not fought to replace an aristocratic aristocracy but to end it! What about the marquee that he made him drag across the mountains? Was his common sense clouded by the mold?

Abel licked his lips, realizing that most officers were in his company.

uncomfortable look. They squirmed nervously and looked towards the window, paying more attention to the poor people than to them. What's the point? This one had a little too much to drink! It's a shame! This one didn't show up on time for picket duty to please the colonel. These brave souls played cards! Oh! These are terrible sins! He felt that the attention of the officers should be on the defense of the settlement and not on harassing their men. The punishments were severe! This one gets fifty lashes! For simply discharging his weapon, this man must stand for five minutes on a sharp picket. This man to be restrained for looking at an officer in disapproval! My fine gentlemen, the enemy was out there! Do not make new men among your own men. He knew that no protest would be of any benefit to him, but it would only lead to ridicule and accusations of being a Tory. This is absurd! They made no sense when they rebuked their men who killed swine, poultry or sheep and burned fence rails for firewood.

The proceedings were finally concluded much to Abel's relief.

Butler stood, and his officers followed him immediately. He stood and his officers immediately followed him.

He bowed slightly and looked at his adjutant, who gave him more papers. He said, "It seems that our docket for the morrow is full as well," and he looked at Abel.

Abel rolled his eyes.

"I'm sure that our fine host will not object to the use of his fine."

Butler stated that he had a large home and was looking forward to the morrow.

His officers made a few cough sounds, which were likely masking.

chuckles.

Butler slammed his foot down on the ground. He said, "Now look here!"

said. All these proceedings follow the Articles of War, and other General Orders that have been published across the American army. It is a surprise to me that disorganized Continental troops could be found violating these rules and orders. If it continues, these courts will follow! It does not state anywhere that separation from the main army invalidates all discipline. We are part the American Army and we will act as such! "Do I need to be clear?"

"Yes sir," they answered in unison. Even Abel Yarington

looked away in shame.

Butler stared at every eye, daring to look at him. He gritted his

His anger was repelled by his teeth. Wyoming will be there, he thought, even though I have to give fifty lashes for every one!

The tension was broken by a rush outside. Everyone

William Stewart, the scout of Colonel Hartley, looked at him. He was surrounded by a staunch officer in a blue regimental. He remained silent, unable to speak or recognize anyone's nod. Butler was handed a dispatch by the scout as he stood up. He said that it was urgent and requested that Butler read it immediately.

Butler rolled his tongue to his cheek. He said, "Very well, these proceedings are closed. But none of you go further." He moved with the paper towards the door. The officers put on their hats, and filed out of the door in silence. They only murmured to each other when the door was closed behind them.

Butler raised his hand towards Yarington.
Abel was a bit confused by the request to vacate his home.

He nevertheless agreed. He entered his kitchen and sat down in a chair. His legs shook angrily on the floor. Stewart stood just outside the door, refusing to be tempted by the already upset man. He cleared his throat and leaned against Yarington's door jam, giving Yarington the majority of the room. He was accompanied by an officer who strode through the room and sat in a chair at a table next to the disgruntled civilian. The man stared at him blankly.

Butler sat down at a great table in the newly vacated main space.

Gently break the wax seal of the dispatch. Before finally unfolding the dispatch, he looked closely at the windows. He began to read it, drawing it near his face:

> September 10, 1778, Colonel Butler, commanding,
> Camp Westmoreland.

"On a thorough consideration of the Indian country, and a

These are my conclusions based on the current circumstances. It is essential that troops from Wyoming, the west branch and this department, make a junction before proceeding against Chemung. This is where, according to my understanding, a large portion of the plunder stolen from our unhappy

Wyoming brethren, as well as a number of Indians, Tories and Tories, are collected. This means that they should approach the town via the Lycoming path that leads to the mouth the Towanda and that troops should sweep the country to Wyoming. This will help our frontiers and instill fear in our enemies. Lieutenant Lemon can provide more details. I have already mentioned some of these details to him.

"I have been told that many of your employees are inclined to the highest degree."

They may also be able to revenge the murders or brothers or fathers and serve their country by going against Indian towns. Captain Kenney will be detained with a Sergeant, ten men from my regiment, and a subaltern. The men who can march are Spalding's or Howe's men. Captain Kenney will take control of the garrison under your immediate supervision. The remainder of my regiment, and the troops at Wyoming, will march from thence to Muncy Fort on Monday next, near Wallis'. All the pack-horses and saddles are required to be brought with them. They are expected to arrive at Fort Muncy on the third or fourth night of their march.

"It will not be possible to tell troops or civilians where they are."

To march to. The militia must be made to march against an Indian town. The garrison must be made aware that the militia has marched to West Branch to help the Indians. The route to Muncy is justifiable; the Tories are fooled. You will do the best you can in the absence of troops. You will be supported by all the troops from this quarter in an emergency. I won't, perhaps, go Chemung. The garrison will continue near Nescopeck. This letter may be sent to Captains Bush, Kenney, and Colonel Dennison. It will also reach Mr. Stewart under strict secrecy. Murray and Mr. Howe have received some intimations. I doubt they will reveal them. The people who are going on this expedition will return in time to plant some Fall grain.

Your most humble and obedient servant

Colonel Thomas Hartley.”
It has, Butler thought. It was a sudden feeling of numbness.

Premonition. It is not clear if this was due to him being uninvited to the expedition or if it warned of a future disaster. He reminded his troops that orders had to be obeyed, and he was right.

He leaned back and rubbed his chin. He complied with the surrender terms

He had a flashback to valley, but he knew they were already violated by both sides. The Indians were in for a surprise. Surprise and lesson. They would be able to learn it well this time. He was certain. It was very secure for him.

Beware Queen Ester, and her betraying band!

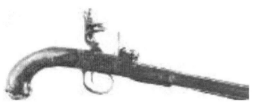

Chapter Twenty

Colonel Hartley watched as the troops slowly made their way to Fort Muncy, with a feeling of hollowness in his heart. Pennsylvania promised five hundred troops. The small number of soldiers milling around the fort didn't bode well for Hartley.

He stood by himself, surrounded by a large tree that spanned the distance between Wallis' stone home and the new fort. He stopped and walked around for a time, looking at the trees between Wallis' stone house and the new fort. He thought they would, he believed. It was not difficult for men with such wisdom and determination to be elected to defend the country to see their vulnerable backdoor. A flood could descend right down to Philadelphia from the southern entrance at Tioga Point of the Iroquois Nation. It has already happened once. It had stopped at Wyoming, thank God. Don't leave the door unlocked! You must close it or put a foot against it.

He rubbed his head, cursing the persistent ague pestering.

him. He pulled his regimental coat around his frame and took a deep inhale. He saw two men coming from the corner of his eyes. He looked at them.

"Colonel," said the taller one, as he threw his hat. "This is Hawkins Boone Captain as I. He is detached here to help in any way possible.

Hartley said "Yes Captain Brady", extending his hand towards Boone. All are welcome, sir. "A clever group of men is assembling here, is it not?"

Brady stated, "Clever," but not great in numbers.

Boone stated that numbers don't necessarily indicate where we are going. "Guts are what matters up there!"

"Yes, thank God, courage doesn't seem to be lacking in this

Hartley stated that men are gathering here.

Boone stated, "Each man with a rifle here in the country is a crack shot."

His extremely long rifle was raised. He could clearly see that it was a foot above his head. "I can't speak for fowling items and musketeers, however."

Hartley winced at Captain Murray's reference to his six-month tenure

Men and his regiment. He stated flatly that he had ordered all rifles not carried to be loaded with swanshot and provided ample cartridges.

Boone stated, "Swan shot, I say." "That's fine. All one has to do is

Point and shoot, anything close will catch the lead. It is great for bush fighting.

Hartley stated, "Well, I'm glad you agree.".
Brady stated, "It's time we taught the Savages a proper lessons."

In the midst of a haunting thought, eyes turn to the sky and look up. Young James must be avenged. James is a finer son than any man has ever had. He will be sorely missed.

Boone said, "Much must be avenged.".
Hartley stated, "We will do everything we can, I promise you both.".
Brady asked, "Then it's true that this force will march upon the Nations?".
Hartley replied, "We will do what we can," pointing a finger at Hartley.

His nose said, "But we must keep our mouths shut. Surprising is the essence of surprise. These are difficult times. One day, a man may be loyal to Congress and the next, he might be loyal to the Crown.

Brady reached for the long knife from his belt with his left hand. He began to draw it.

He raised the long blade to his neck. He said, his eyes ablaze with purpose, "If I know of any such,".

Hartley's eyes widen at Hartley's gesture. These men were grim.

frontier meant business. They were both Tory or savage. He felt less concerned about numbers, perhaps spirit was more important than number. One of his men was worth three times as much as the enemy.

All their attention was drawn to a call from the fort. Captain Walker

Hartley waved at him, and then to the small, muscular man standing beside him. Hartley replied by raising his hand. Hartley was immediately in his sights as the man nodded at Walker.

Boone, who was cocking his head, said "Well, we'll just be about our business."

Head to Brady. Before turning around and walking towards the fort, they touched the brims on their hats. They were ignored by the little man, who continued to march past them, seemingly determined to reach the colonel.

The man said "Herr Colonel", shifting his rifle to the left. He reached into his pocket and pulled out a folded piece of paper. He carefully unfolded it and presented it to the colonel.

Hartley took out the paper and began to read it. He was slightly relieved that he had found it.

There will not be another dispatch from a commander of militia regretting his inability at present to answer his call.

He read the commission and said "Ensign Fox", It is good to see you.

Do you have word for your regiment?

Fox stated, "Nien ich here on my own account," "Krieg has

They all. Der wildens, der Tories! They march to this spot, I believe. Ich join you. Ich will fight!"

Hartley stated, "It's good to have you." Hartley said, "As yet your regiment."

Although they have yet to arrive, I do hope that they will soon.

Fox exclaimed, "Ja Colonel, they'll, I know it to be true," lifting

His rifle was used to rub the stock. "Fine shot, I am, der wildens a took me twice, they won't again!"

Walker: "This man is very knowledgeable about the upriver region."

It was as if it had come from nothing.

Hartley gave the paper back to the Palatine German with a smart nod.

He took it gently and lowered his rifle to the floor.

The prized paper was meticulously folded. He smiled proudly and placed the paper back in its desired place in his bag.

Walker stated that Walker has property around the Towanda Creek. "He

He knows Ester's village as well as Sheshecunnunk and Tioga as well as the Queen. This knowledge could prove to be invaluable."

Hartley stared at Walker for a moment. Hartley glared at Walker for a moment.

Through gritted teeth, it "may not, also."

Walker ignored the hint and remained silent. Walker was puzzled by the reason.

When rumors spread throughout the valley, colonel remained firm in his resolve. It didn't take long to understand the purpose of this rendezvous. He was able to keep his mouth shut, even though he had doubts about whether the Dutchman understood the significance of the matter. He was a staunch patriot and a friend of the Crown, but he had also been a loyal patriot.

Fox smiled, "I'se See About Mien Interests," Fox said.

His face. "Das burned, I bet. Barn, cabin, and all."

Walker stated, "This war is hell for us all.".
Hartley said, "Yes, and hell has ears perked just for such information."

said.

Walker moved his lips and rubbed his chin.

"Anyway Ensign Fox, we are glad to have you. Find a place to settle."

Hartley looked up at the yellow, orange and crimson leaves that dotted the trees around him and said "I will wait for orders." "I promise you will not have to wait for long."

Walker waited for the German to walk well beyond earshot before he spoke.

Before speaking again. "We only have eighty-four men here as of yet. We have the finest powder I've ever seen and many of these men are excellent shots. There are enough barrels of whiskey and flour to last us for two weeks, sir.

Hartley muted that he was eighty-four from the five hundred promised or

Even the four hundred that he thought he required for a proper expedition. It was necessary to make do, but it seemed absurd. He clenched one fist and gritted his teeth to combat the doubts that plagued him. Those damn politicians. It's great to have commanders on the field, but what good is it if they are managed and controlled by people far away from the work, hands that are not stained by sweat, blood, and tears? General Wayne had said to him that men with his vision could be as effective on the floor as they were in the field. The general's insight was something he reflected on, and he thought about it again. Congress needed men with good horse sense.

He looked at Walker, who was pacing about a great tree. It took a full

There are twenty steps that can be taken to control the object's circumference. He thought of Philadelphia's many trees as he admired each branch. Before approaching Walker again, he carefully surveyed the scene. He said, "Look at it man," and raised his arms against the massive girth of the majestic elm. It alone could build a beautiful house with plenty of board feet! Take a look around! He looked around. He kicked the ground with his feet and scratched a spot in its fertile soil.

Walker stated, "It's a rich country, sir.".

Hartley stated, "Yes, rich and in contention with three great powers." Hartley said that there is more to this than just a foray against brazen savages. Empires must be built and won. Wyoming is not forgotten, You will find great minds working on this issue, I assure you. We risk losing vast stretches of land if we don't settle this conflict now. Canada's borders will be the Hudson, Sunbury, and possibly Carlisle. This land is too important for America. If we want to see peace, we must conquer the Six Nations, our great enemy to the north. It is essential to any expansion of our fledgling country to the west or north.

Walker was silent and let the colonel vent their frustrations.

"Colonel Butler, Fourth Pennsylvania, is set to march at

This is Morgan's riflemen. We will meet at Tioga Point to teach Brant, Butler and the Johnsons a valuable lesson that they won't soon forget. What about Brant? Are you thinking of Brant? Eightyfour men are not enough. Where are Spalding and Bush? We might have a chance with their help, but without them it will be futile. These men are too good for me. Wallis and Smith, together with that man Smith," he said, mumbling to himself, ashamed of having revealed his deepest thoughts.

Walker said "I believe," and then added, "that our good people, this intelligent."

"Body of men will be asking themselves where the devil has gone to their colonel."

Hartley said, "Yes, I think they will."

He lowered his head and regained his composure. He said, "Thanks Captain!".
Walker smiled a little. "Come sir, there!"

The question of who will rule over this vast land is still to be resolved. It will be done by Americans, I can assure you. This is where I feel God's hand."

"What does Doctor Franklin say?" God is good to those who help themselves?" Hartley asked.

Walker nodded his head.

Two men entered a vast clearing of five hundred.

Yards were all around the fort's palisades. Both marched spiritedly towards the bustling fort and accelerated their steps when they heard the sounds of martial music and cheering.

The column marched in a smart manner into the clearing. Two mounted men

Both sat in their vans, one wearing a smart blue regimental coat and white facings, the other wearing a double-breasted brown coat with red sleeves and red collar. They sat in the saddle high, saluting each other and doffing their hats. They were joined by four musicians who marched quickly in front of them, performing lively tunes. They were followed by a wide variety of men, some ragged and shabby, but they looked smart nonetheless.

They were beaming with joy at every face they met. Rifles

The cannons blazed into the air. Cannons boomed. The men were jovial when the fearful air rose above them.

Walker stated, "They bring great spirit with them," Hartley said, and stopped just before the column's front.

Hartley: "To say nothing, my good Captain.

said. He watched as the captains brought their horses to a halt and ordered their men's column to stop.

Captain Spalding exclaimed, "Colonel Hartley!" He took off his hat.

He swept it in a wide arc towards the column of men ahead. "Wyoming is here, sir!"

Hartley stated, "Indeed it has Captain." Hartley said, "Indeed it has!"

much welcomed! You are very welcome sir!

Chapter Twenty-One

Colonel Hartley lay down nervously, his mind occupied by the constant humming and calling of the forest. Are they really the forest creatures calling? Or were they just pretenders corrupting the calls to their own evil ends? What would they do? He swore to protect innocent civilians or one of his soldiers? He swore to protect all of them.

A second eerie sound was heard in the night. This sent chills racing.

His spine. He tossed his blanket aside and searched in the dark for his boots, until he heard the sentry calling. The sendry helped him to his bed. He wondered aloud, "Will it never end?" It was only a matter of time before the enemy was put in his place and subjugated. But how? But how can one fight the night and its tyrants? The enemy was bolder and uttered more war-cries in the dark of the night over the last few nights. Is it just braggadocio from a soldier of a passing battle party or affirmation that they saw everything in the fort? These thoughts rattled his brain, making it a mental torture that kept him up at night. It was no wonder that his weak body was plagued by the ague. He would wake up in the middle of the night with war cries, just as he was drifting off to sleep. It was a mystery to him. Could it have been a sign or pure chance?

He pulled up his blanket and stared out of the window at the darkness.

Night, realizing that there would never be another night of sleep. He waited, as he had done every night since late, for the gentle glow that dawn would bring. How did he greet the day?

Two days ago, the rest of his regiment and Wyoming were dissolved.

The troops arrived. He knew that no one else had answered his call and would have to use the tools he had. It was urgent to make a decision. Or March?

A faint glimmering of like was visible through the widow.

The stone wall. He quickly found his boots and tossed his blanket aside. He surveyed his troops today. He would make a decision today, because the season was getting late, and soon the majority of the men would need to return to the fields to harvest the late harvest. This is as important as dealing the IndianTory threat. It was imperative that the grain be harvested, and that the Indian and Tory threat be addressed. He had half of the troops needed to launch an effective punitive operation against the enemy. Half the troops, half of the chance of success. Can the frontier withstand another defeat? A victory, even if small, could do more to help the frontier's faltering frontier than any other thing. The victory could also encourage more settlers to return the Susquehanna frontier. More settlers means more security for the nation and the frontier. Yes, he must get out of his way, now!

His mind was tangled up in anxious thoughts when he heard a knock at the door. Wallis' servant called him as if he had been waiting outside the door all night. Is he watching him or is he just anxious? He replied, "Yes, I am up.".

The servant spoke from the other side of his door, "Fine sir." "I've

fetched some fresh milk. I'll be there waiting for you."

He said, "I'm certain you will," under his breath.

He quickly washed his face in a basin and then shaved. He donned and

Straightening his regimental jacket, he opened the door latch and half-expected the servant to greet him. He looked down at the empty hallway and sighed before making his way down. A bowl of fresh milk and a loaf bread sat on a kitchen table. He sat down, and passed his hat to the always-waiting servant.

The great smile that spans the black reveals white teeth

man's face. He bows and retreats to the stairway. "Master Wallis

He explained that he wanted to know when guests rose. Hartley waved his hand, saying "I'll fetch he.".

The servant replied, "No sir." "He's a want'n to know and the master."

He does what he wants, and he gets it!"

Hartley said "Very well," after putting a piece of bread in the grater.

The bowl contained milk. He picked up the spoon, but then dropped it. He suddenly lost appetite. Wallis grumbled down the hall, and a drum roll was heard from the fort. In the wakefulness and grogginess from being awakened so early, Hartley was showing a little of his true colors. Hartley thought. Hartley thought.

Before his host, he ate several heaping spoonfuls of milk and bread.

Wallis rose and wished to go about his business unaffected by Wallis. Wallis seemed to be more interested in the operations of his command over time.

Hartley would have stayed behind the walls of Fort Wallis if Wallis had not gained the trust of John Dickinson and Benjamin Rush. Hartley could then observe the clever landowner from safety at arm's reach. To do so now would be an insult to Wallis and to all those who had his confidence. He speculated that they might have known more about the man than he. He would smile and accept his advice with politeness, while also offering his compliments with thinly disguised compliments.

He called the hallway and said, "I have business to attend too."

Waiting for a reply before donning his hat, and walking out of the door. "I am sorry for any inconvenience."

He was greeted by the bright sun. He reached out to protect his eyes with his hand.

Pay attention to the surroundings. He marched towards the fort after nodding to a saluting sendry.

Spalding, Bush, and Captain Walker greeted him at his gate.

The fort. After cordial salutations, they all turned and looked around at the troops. All along the parade ground, fires blazed. Frames of logs were used as foundations for barracks and other buildings. Men rose from the frames. Everyone seemed excited and eager to get up. There were no grumbles or complaints, like they did in any other fatigue camp Hartley ever experienced. It was a pleasant surprise. He smiled at the officers and expressed his appreciation to them.

Bush straightened his fine uniform, saying "A fine bunch they are." Hartley observed that he looked odd among the other ragged, threadbare men around him. But he did it every day. The man was able to repair his uniform and maintain it in a perfect state, even though he took part in the activities of his colleagues. He was a bit of a dandy but a great commander of troops. He wouldn't trade his man for another officer of the same rank.

Bush was looked at by all three officers, who seemed to be silently staring at each other.

Hartley shares Hartley's assessment of the man.

Bush raised an eyebrow in their direction.

Hartley stated, "None is more fine than the officers that lead them."

Breaking the uneasy air. "I have assembled an intelligent body of men, am I not?"

"Each man-jack is equal to thrice your enemy," I dare to say.

sir," Spalding said.
"Yes, no doubt," Hartley said.

Bush asked, "Are you to march soon Colonel?".

Hartley told Walker, "I am thinking about the matter.".
Walker nodded.
Bush stated, "I pity any wild this lot encounters sir", and "be he."

Blue-eyed, or what? Yes, sir! Yes, sir!

Hartley replied, "Yes." Hartley said, "Let the men eat first and then assemble them."

review."

All the captains replied "Yes sir", at once. They cleverly turned

They marched toward their troops wearing cocksures and smiling reassuring smiles.

Hartley was open to a few nods and stares as he acknowledged them.

He walked around the fort. He climbed up to a platform at the wall and politely nodded to the men. But he was eager to get away from their curious eyes. He lowered his hands to the wall and stared blankly at it, his thoughts lost.

He turned only when the drum beat assembly was over. He was not clapping his hands.

He raised his hands and gazed at the well-assembled ranks. Each man stood straight and stern with his eyes fixed on the front, and each firelock sat straight on a shoulder. He paused for a moment and slowly began to climb down the ladder. He stepped onto the ladder and faced the straight ranks.

Bush raised his sword to his face, then lowered it to his chest.

salute. The salute was quickly adopted by the other officers.

Hartley marched through the ranks instantly, stopping just now

Then, he was to confront a few men. One particular man caught his attention. His eyes were a reflection of his character and stood out above the rags covering him. His beaver-skin hat was ill-fitted on his head. The brim of the hat was covered in disorganized clumps that dangled all over. His well-worn, short brown coat was covered in bits of red hair that were soiled and faded. His right shoulder was adorned with a frayed shoulder strap. His chest was stuffed with pride, as a brown strap crossed his chest. The one strap held a cartridge box, while the other had a sheath that contained a cutlass. Each strap was well worn and the knot at its halfway point tied it. His thighs were covered in frayed and worn breeches that were once white. Below them, bare legs were exposed. Many thorns had scratched and cut his legs. He wore buckleless shoes. The right shoe was bound by a tied rag, while the toes extended from the front of his left shoe.

Hartley tried to keep the shock away from his face but it was too much for him.

The curious look in the eyes of the soldier was a clear sign. The soldier replied, "Don't worry Colonel", forgoing military discipline in favor of the moment. He looked directly into the eyes of the colonel. "We are all ready for march, if you're willing to lead us all. We will make you proud. Yes sir, we will.

Hartley stated, "You already have," and he looked down at the entire thing.

line. "You all have."
The soldier was again in his sights, but he only saw him once more.

His eyes were full of courage and a call for duty, and his soldier's eyes reflected back at him. Where can we find such men? Hartley wondered to himself. These men, mutilated and dressed in rags clamored for the march and a fight against the enemy. They may have been clothed in rags, but their patriotic spirit was what fed them. As he stared into those eyes, all doubt was gone from his mind. March we must!

He said, "Captain Bush!" and stepped back from the Wyoming soldier. Prepare for the march! We will leave at the first light of the morning! Four days of rations are required. Then, send the Indian and Tory rats to hell!

The troops immediately let out a roar of laughter.

From the officers. He raised his head and marched back towards Wallis' house, sure that he and his brave men would be able to withstand the hardships of the march as well as the inevitable battle ahead.

Chapter Twenty-Two

The night was lit by great fires, which cast many shadows against Fort Muncy's tall walls. Since Colonel Hartley's march yesterday morning, no one had slept more than a few minutes. No one complained. Nobody slowed down. They waited too long to have this chance. They would fight the war on the frontier with the same rigor as those fighting the British regulars. For they knew that not only was their country dependent upon it but also their lives and their prosperity.

Colonel Hartley walked up-and-down a line pack-horses.

Each one was examined by the light of a burning pine needle held by a private, He stopped now and again to tug at the straps that held the barrels and the packs tight to the horses' backs. He gently patted the horse's rump. "Good job to everyone." He glanced over at the officer who was watching him. "All is well Captain Sweeney. Is it not?"

Sweeney replied, "Oh, yes sir." "We have whiskey and flour."

a good twelve days!"

Hartley moved past him to reach one of the smaller kitchens.

fires dotting the ground. He looked down to flat hot rocks sizzling with flour cakes mixed with potash. "Plenty of boiled beef and ash cake for all," he said, walking over to another group preparing for the march.

An officer saluted, "We are ready Colonel", and raised his rifle. He raised his rifle and proudly declared, "Any savage falling' under these sights shall die his last!"

In the wake of the boast, huzzas erupted.

Hartley stated, "I do indeed possess the best powder-markmen I ever seen!" Hartley saluted many noggins.

Hartley stated, "But take it easy on the whiskey lads." Hartley said, "For it."

It doesn't have to be for the entire duration of your trip. It's important to be smart about it. We will march soon so if you want to catch a wink, do it now! Once we are done, it will be with blankets at the thump, and at the long trot.

He was answered by another huzza from his energetic group of men. He

Simon Spalding smiled at them and raised his head in salute.

Hartley raised his hands and ran off to other areas of the camp.

He felt more inspired by the growing spirit among the men, the more he spoke with them.

Spalding told a lieutenant next to him, "There's an excellent man."

He was a great man. He was a great soldier during the Canadian campaign. He also has General Washington's ears. He considers his Excellency part of his 'family,' which he refers to those who are close to him.

"Yes, I believe Congress has made the right decision placing him."

here," Lieutenant Jenkins said.
Spalding might see a hint in Jenkins' eyes, despite his seemingly unrelenting support.

words. He said, "It is a hell of war, it's, not for land, or for some faraway sovereign, but for an idea." An ideal is one in which a man can be treated according to his own standards and not the way his father was. This war, this brave new step forwards requires a special breed, one who steps up when necessary but fades to the background when it is not. Like Captain Ransom and Durkee, I believe Mr. Hartley is a member of this special breed.

Jenkins stated, "That's for certain.".
"This country, this new land, founded on ideals treads on shaky

Spalding stated that ground is a new ground that has only been walked a handful of times in human history." "Beginning on such unstable ground, we have little resources, so we must make do with the things we have and trust Providence will bless and shine upon our great endeavor."

Jenkins stared in awe at Jenkins. He said, "You've been thinking about this,"

said. "Have you not?"
"Aye, through many marches on the cool summer grass and upon

The hard, frozen ground of winter. It is not right to take all the responsibility on one's own, but it is better to trust that others will take over. God is with us, regardless of what happened at Wyoming. To grow, one must endure, and we certainly have had our fair share. We are now at the forefront of a new direction.

Jenkins glanced down at his right hand. Jenkins rubbed the area.

He did the same thing he did last year when he was taken prisoner to Niagara. He placed it where Beth last held it for him. He felt the warmth of her eyes as he rubbed it on his cheek. When he touched her hand, he still felt the warmth from her heart. It had supported him through the dark, terrible hole in Fort Niagara's floor and throughout his journey through the wilderness. It would also sustain him now.

Spalding was immediately aware of Spalding's odd behavior after he met him.

The late battle. He was not wrong. Wyoming was touched by the beauty of Bethiah Kinsen's work. We could not survive without love, but what could? He turned away, pretending to not notice his actions.

Jenkins said, "For Beth it's that I fight," under his breath. "And

for everyone's Beth."

Spalding was puzzled by the comment. He remembered his grandfather's.

Own wife and children. He said, "You are to keep a watch on the country through whom we pass, and noting everything you can." "I am here, as you all know, in more than the capacity of Captain Wyoming Rangers, as His Excellency has been known for calling us, but also as a military advisor."

Jenkins stopped rubbing his hands. A man like Colonel Hartley's

Experience is a great source of advice. However, it's more useful to have it.

Spalding, looking out from the corner, said that "More is at Play here."

His young lieutenant was looking into his eyes. "After this expedition, either you or me will be called to headquarters. We will then brief His Excellency about all that we saw on the expedition. I'm sure Colonel Hartley will also do this. His Excellency needs a frontiersman's view of things. One who is knowledgeable about the land. One who can walk it in both war and peace. One who can see the enemy from a distance." He glanced down at the flames in front of him. "That's why it will likely be you who reports to General Washington. The country is in a delicate balance, with a large portion of it still unresolved. It should be part of our country, not the bloody Crown. You have been told everything you need to know. At the moment, it is an order. Remember this: Remember where they fight and how you beat them.

Jenkins nodded and looked over at him. He said, "I will, sir.".
Spalding stated, "I know you will," and "you're a good man."

They extended a hand to the throngs of troops. "Now let's prepare these men for march, for their fathers, mothers and sons are in our charge. After all the dust has settled, we will return them safe and sound. Let us now be focused on our duties and trust Providence to guide us through this valley.

Chapter Twenty-Three

Colonel Hartley took his watch from his waistcoat pocket and kept it safe. It was an important and rare prize on frontier. He squinted in the light of the firelight to read the hands. It was painfully obvious that he was being watched by so many eager people. It was four o'clock in morning. Although the sun was still illuminating the horizon, the men in his command demanded that they move now. He took it as a sign and raised his hand shouting "forward!"

The men made the first step with perfect cadence and wailed an off the

Cuff song with a chorus that sounded like "Nothing like Grog" They marched proudly behind their officers, not a single eye looking back at the fort. All eyes gazed forward, towards the mountains and its protective forest, in an effort to teach those who lived there a lesson they would never forget. It had to be done.

The sun rose from their front, gracing the mountains with a heavenly glow.

light. With no difficulty, lively footsteps swept across the Loyalsock creek ford. Spirited eyes gazed to one another, and the raindrops falling from the darkening skies.

Hartley called Hartley back and said, "Close up!" "Flankers tighten up! Be

To give spirited huzzas, he rode back along his line. He nodded at the men's yells and ordered them to be smart and keep close to the others. To his dismay, the line actually slowed down rather than accelerating to his words.

He instantly turned and galloped to the front.

Robert Covenhoven and a few Wyomingites eager to help

scouts, met him. "No worries," Covenhoven said. "It's only here where the trail cuts north, it gets a bit rough. But we'll get through it," Covenhoven said.

Hartley looked ahead, and down into the valley into which the trail led.

led. The wind blew cattails in the wind, showing intermittent water spots. He looked back at Covenhoven. He asked, "A swamp?".

Colonel Covenhoven stated, "Just a little bit of a wade suffices." "These

It's not difficult for men to get through it. It's nothing compared to what lies ahead. Although the Sheshequin Path is not for everyone, it is one of our favorite routes at this point.

Hartley lifted his spyglass up to his eye and gazed through the rain.

The other side of the swamp. Once it had passed through a large amount of rocks, the trail rose steeply to dense trees. He asked, "What's that?" "Rocks?"

Covenhoven stated, "It's all the God's hand made, Colonel." "We will get through with his help.

He is only seven miles from the Fort and his Scouts are already seeking him

The Lord's help. The season came too late. He was astonished to hear from his Scouts about the difficulties involved in using the Wyalusing Path. He licked his lips. He said, "Very well." "Let us continue until dark."

"We'll be fine sir, because with this lot one is just as tough as the

"Next," he was assured by one of the men.

He dismounted and led his horse into the swamp. Already

Men tugged on the mud. With each step through the bog, suckling sounds filled the air. In a few places, even his horse groaned and stumbled in frustration. He eventually led his horse to solid ground amid the rocks, and stood watching as the men struggled past. He was surprised to find that not one complaint and only encouraging words drifted through his ranks. A quick scold was enough to put an end to the groan that did arise. His pride was heightened by the sight of the rain-soaked, struggling men who were enduring the hardships without any hint of ridicule. He thought these men were a vicious bunch and he was right.

They made it through the swamp to reach dense hemlocks but they were not able to stop them.

The drenching rains brought little relief. There were few voices along the trail because despite all the hardships everyone knew to remain silent, even without any word from their officers. They heard the dense shadows speak to them, a warning that was deeper than any of their officers. A few fell on the increasingly muddy trail and lost their feet, but they quickly recovered their footing.

Slowly, the day turned into night. Dripping branches from the trees were a reminder of their fate.

The deluge of the heavens added to the steady stream of water that fell on the column. Finally, the column came to a stop atop a hill carefully chosen.

Walker reported to his soaked, "This'll work fine sir."

colonel. "It's best for us to be high so that we can keep an eye out down below. Besides, they won't expect us to camp here."

Hartley said, "Very well Captain," plopping down from his chair.

saddle. His boots touched the ground and a torrent of water surged up the top.

Walker stated, "You'd be best to remove them for the night.". Hartley almost laughed as he shook his head. Hartley shook his head, almost chuckling.

Take them to the creek to dry, and you'll be amazed at how humid it is up there.

Walker was a bit irritated by the colonel's attempts at humor. "We'll

To make a hut, you can use a few branches to create a shelter.

"Talk about impossible, it would have to be this expedition and desire

Hartley declared, while slapping his horse's back. His face was splattered with water. He asked, "Do the Iroquois own a navy?".
Walker smiled as he raised his head above his wide, slouchy hat.

stretching across his face.
Hartley approached Hartley and placed his hand on his shoulder. Hartley said, "Come, my dear man, we will partake in whiskey, no chill could stand against it.".
Walker stated, "Boiled beef and fire cake, whiskey," after he had finished his

Commander into a dense grove full of hemlock boughs. "It's a proper campaign isn't it?"

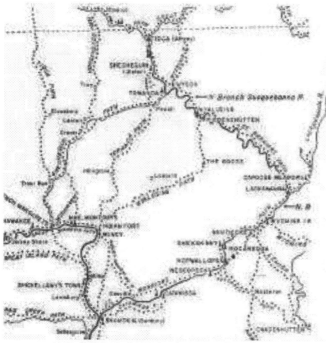
A map showing Indian Paths along Susquehanna River

Chapter Twenty-Four

In the damp forest, the dull sound of axes was heard. The torrents of rain had soaked the men who were willing to give up their axes. But they ignored it and continued swinging their axes in fury. The path had to be cleared.

Hartley exclaimed, "The axe seems just as important as the rifle" as he watched the men hammer away at the underbrush and fallen trees blocking the trail. Hartley reached into his bag and pulled out an ash cake. He rushed to put it in his mouth before the rain stopped. He ate the cake and looked back at the men huddled in wait for the path to clear. He felt a moment of frustration, but it was not enough. He said, "Fate has ordained that" he would go to war against the savages in America instead of the British to an officer who was walking beside him.

> The officer quickly replied, "Yes, but it's a war that must be fought."

countered.

> Hartley dipped his head and said "It's true Captain Stoddert."

Let a steady stream water flow from his hat. "You must feel at home, because you are fond of the sea."

> Stoddert, staring at the stillness, said "I've never seen such rainfall."

Men held their weapons close to their bodies to protect themselves from the rain. Some wrapped leather around the locks. Some covered the locks with leather bits, while others used bits of their ragged clothes that they ripped off their backs. They didn't raise a complaint or murmur.

> Hartley observed Stoddert's words and said "But with men like these."

Gaze, "it's a pleasure to command. If they are properly trained, I believe they can do anything. Beware of Brant and Ester."

> Spalding, approaching from the rear, said that "they well should at that."

rear. "This is a new kind of war Colonel, but it's still more brutal than any action between civilized men. Don't listen to the old British stories about humanity. It seems that it is extinct out here. The boys I lead expect nothing and will not give anything. Isn't there a hidden curse in the stories about hell that will destroy those who use such tools to create tyranny?

Hartley was shocked by the mention of British officials holding

Their native allies kept them on the leash. These Wyomingans were more hateful of them than other people who had been hurt by their actions. He thought that they were a terrible lot. He only wished that he could stop their wrath after they had encountered the enemy. For with wrath came injustice which corrupted both the aggressor and the avenger.

Spalding stated, appearing to make sense of the words: "They are good men until the last."

Hartley's concern, and "shall follow the orders of them placed above them," Stoddert stated.

All eyes were drawn to the sound of a call from the front. Many of the

The axmen raised their hands and motioned them forward, while they eagerly moved on to the next group. They quickly attacked the next dense mass of brush.

Hartley asked, "Will it never end?".
Spalding urged the men who were passing by to "At Tioga Point it'll," Spalding stated.

close up and advance.
Covenhoven appeared suddenly from the brush to the side of the

trail. He appeared as an apparition, appearing out of nowhere. They all shuddered for a moment. Spalding's rifle was quickly lower, but he swung at Spalding.

He warned, "I'd keep an eye on it if you were me, scout.".
Covenhoven nodded and walked quickly towards Hartley.

Hartley nervously wiped the crease of his forehead and stood by the side.

he recalled with great joy how quickly anyone could be seen from the dense forest surrounding them. He thought it was a different war.

Covenhoven stated, "No worries, I have scouts three thick on

each flank. Hartley stated, "They will not let their eyes go, Colonel."
"But what about this trail?" Hartley said. They began to trundle up the trail.

Covenhoven pointed out that the Lycoming is only a mile up the trail. From there, we'll follow the trail up to the Towanda and then it will be Indian country." He snapped a branch in his face. His cheek immediately became reddened. It's hard going, I admit, but this path hasn't been used except infrequently in recent years. They won't expect us."

Stoddert stated, "I can see why," Stoddert explained. He was referring to a slippery root that sent him.

He stumbled to the muddy ground. He gasped and grabbed the moss-covered, saturated log in front of him. He lost his grip on the moss and fell to the ground. Hartley and the Scout helped him get to his feet.

Nennies frustrated by Carberry's horse filing past ripped their eyes.

them.

Stoddert said, "I pity my horse," and rose to his feet.

Covenhoven stated, "I pity them Iroquois encounters," and "I feel

There will be no quarter."

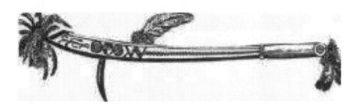

Chapter Twenty-Five

They heard the sound of water rushing past their ears before they saw the creek below. They walked down the narrow path to the clearing at the bank of the raging water. The torrent raged and no one spoke. They were unable to see clearly due to the torrential rains and resorted to using their other senses, including hearing, to warn of dangers. Indian threats.

They parted ways after a movement at the back of their line caused them to make

Their colonel was on his way. Hartley walked to the bank and looked down on one side of the stream, then the other. He asked, "The Lycoming creek?" "What people call a creek, would be a small river for me."

Covenhoven declared, "None of these land's been cleared," and slapped the wet.

Buckskin holding onto his mud-caked body. "Moss and dead leaves, old rotten woods, all of them hold the water, just like this accursed buckskin. It makes it run higher on cleared farmland as close to York and Lancaster." He looked at the stream and shook his head. "With these rains, it'll play hell upon our advance.

It scared me. The trail is narrow and it leads to this place.

Hartley replied, "Yes," rubbing his hands under his brim.

soaked hat. "This is where it takes you. Do you know of any better fording spots?

Covenhoven stated, "I am afraid that what you see is what it will be, sir.".
Hartley stated, "Well, blast that, it shall not hinder us," Hartley said, "If the savage..."

"If Tory can manage this trail," he said, gesturing to the horsemen standing behind him. Captain Carberry, send your horsemen downstream to capture any men swept away by these wild waters. Keep your cartridge boxes and horns as high as possible, rest of you! The tallest men should be at the front, where they can lock arms and form an iron chain that crosses the river. All the others will follow it! Let's get on with it! Right away!"

Horsemen quickly reacted and charged down the trail. Men

They parted to make room for them, while fixing their cartridge boxes and powder horns to their bayonet muskets. Some riflemen quickly cut down small tree limbs and saplings in order to raise their powder horns high above their heads.

Carberry drove his horse straight into the brown without hesitation

water. It almost rolled over at first before it regained its footing and rose again. Carberry held the reins in one arm and balanced his rifle with the other. His horse's flanks were sprayed with white water. It was a fine horse, and stood with the same zeal as its master.

Carberry called his horsemen to the bank, "Come now!".
"Let's go! "The water is fine!"

They followed their leader into the torrent. They did not know what to do.

They were only a few feet from each other when they fell into the water.

Carberry waved his hand and whistled at those who waited on the bank, waving his hands.

In the air. "Come on, let's move!"

Taller men fell into the rapids. They were initially hesitant.

The bottom fell, but the men soon formed a line that stretched from one bank of the river to another. The strongest men were in the middle, and water rushed against their chests and into the pits. They made powerful oaths to the Indians and Tories, and spat out brown water.

Hartley gazed at the wide-eyed eyes that were watching him and stepped into the ground.

The water came first. He plodded slowly along the line of men, fighting against the current. He was pushed against the current by the water, but he continued to walk along the line, always mindful of the ranks and files behind him. Many of them were half a foot shorter than his average height. He let out a sigh and reached the safety of the bank.

Colonel, you shouldn't have done it," Covenhoven moaned.

He is behind him. "We haven't scouted out the bank yet. You're lucky to still have your hair!" "Blast it!"

Hartley turned to offer his hand to the bank and said "I".

The scout said, "I intend to keep my hair well into older age, thank you." He raised the man from the water and immediately lowered his hand to assist the next one. He said, "Don't worry too much about me," and he turned briefly to the Scout. "Now, be focused on your business!"

"Woe to any Iroquois who run up against that obstinate demi-god!"

One of the scouts who had been following Covenhoven's trail stated that he was not sure.

Covenhoven replied, "Just the kind we need for this company.". Both men rolled up the brims of their wet slouch caps.

Scanning the trees around you. Covenhoven stated, "Damn that luckless fool who would be out there in this weather anyhow." "Be he friend, or foe."

Another scout nodded, his head drenched from sweating down a great deal.

He takes a sip from his canteen.

He said, "Amen to it," and passed the canteen to Covenhoven. "Amen to this."

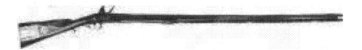

Chapter Twenty-Six

They rose at the first light, drank copious amounts whiskey, and continued up the narrow trail through the valley. The Lycoming Creek's hairpin turns proved difficult enough for even the most patient of men to negotiate. In some areas, wild vines were hanging from every tree. They were surrounded by tangled wild vines that hung from every tree. Lycoming Creek roared and hissed all around them, increasing their dread at the prospect of being forced to ford it again.

Colonel Hartley finally pulls a long, sticky vine from under his foot.

He ordered a stop. He sat on top of a large, moss-covered and soaked boulder while he waited for his officers and scouts to get to him.

They walked up the rock and circled it, some kneeling at its feet.

While others moved around it. They were all silent and thought nothing of their frustrations. They silently looked ahead at the trail, which, to their dismay crossed over the raging water again. If they crossed it, it would be their seventh attempt! Others gazed up at the bizarre conical-shaped hills around them. The steep slopes of their steep faces were covered in half-rotten logs and slippery rocks. They waited for the colonel's words to speak, but the terrain was too frightening for them.

Hartley lifted his hat to see the water and said "Look at that damn thing!"

He slapped it against his thigh. He felt the rain pour down on his face and he squinted against it. He screamed, "Damn it!" and he threw his soaked hat back on his head. "What about these damn mountains!" They look more like anthills than any mountain I have ever seen. We should try to climb their steep faces, not fight those damn waters again.

His logic was unquestioned by anyone. They turned to the exhausted

Men lying in the mud, on rocks, fallen logs or any other place that offers a break from their difficult trek.

Hartley stated that the closer we are to the creek's head, the better. It has diminished some in force, but it will be damned if it is again. Not this day at all.

In their exhausted state, his officers and scouts were silent.

Hartley stated, "Then it is up the damn anthill mountain," his mind.

He flashes back to the terrible trip to Canada that he made just two years ago.

He thought that it was not worth the pain of this horrible march in comparison to the hellish trail. He thought, but they had to keep going. He dropped from the boulder and waved his frustrated hand at the hill in front of them. He said, "Let's get it done," and looked up at the dark sky above.

"Daylight's burning, I believe, if we have not abandoned the sun too," he said. A few laughs answered his attempts at humor.

He said, "Ester's warriors will wait if the sun's radiation is not."

With a serious look. "So let's be smart and alert. There may be more dangers than the accursed rattlesnakes that infest this land behind every rock. Personally, I would take one of these vile serpents over any savage. At least, rattlesnakes will give you warning before they strike!

The men replied to their questions in a single file and in good order.

They were exhausted and pushed up the mountainside by their fellow officers. The officers agreed that the mountainside was better than the Lycoming's infernal and raging waters. The water seemed to boil at the mercy of nature's fury.

Hartley: "This should be a surprise to the enemy!"

He exclaimed as he watched his men slide against the muddy.

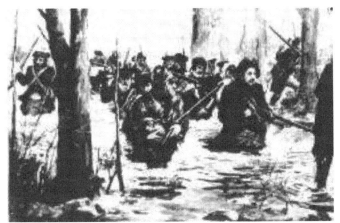

Muddy black soil and wet stones on the side. "It has been a bit of a one for me to be honest."

An anonymous voice said, "Nothing gained from nothing ventured."

commented from the ranks.

"Oh, the gain will be quite substantial, I promise that."

Covenhoven responded to the call. "Keep your powder dry, and your flints clean. You never know when the savages might supply you with sport." Another call came from the ranks.

"Remember Wyoming! It was quickly answered.

Each person's tired lungs echoed the two calls. The words faded

The last man disappeared around the mountain. Their exhausted ranks now sat silently. Their dark enemy's land was silent. Silence that is tinged by despair.

A few people in the ranks saw the despair and passed along encouraging words. The despair soon subsided under the influence of their determination and thirst for revenge.

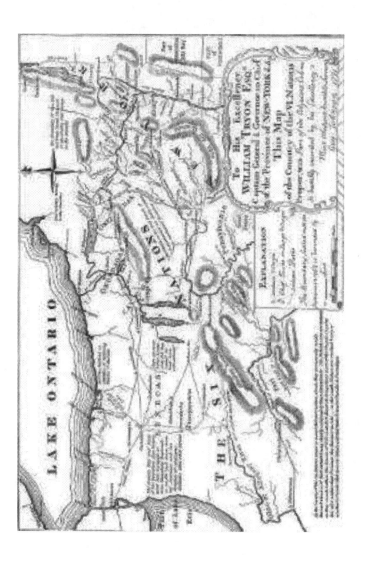

Chapter Twenty-Seven

Ester's village was cloaked in the morning sun. A few Wyoming sheep were captured and bleated in still air. From the plain to the west, bellowing cows answered. Beyond the sun's rays, the shadows of the tall trees that surrounded the mountains all around the village glowed across the face the Susquehanna River. The riverbanks were lined with great overshadowing trees, their branches reaching down to the river's surface as if they were drinking from its waters. There were only a few bare spots between the trees. These were mainly round fields of corn and canoe landings. A few pine bough huts were scattered along the riverbank at one of the landings.

One of the children was ragged and bare-skinny.

Their light skin shining in the morning sun shines through the huts. The boys knelt next to a smoldering flame, one of them carefully placing logs on it. The boys watched as a third child, in a filthy and torn dress, moved slowly towards the village, while the other two boys sat nearby.

None of her brothers protested the gnawing feeling inside the

They were savagely hungry. They did however look at the blanket that was hanging above the door of the hut with some apprehension. They waited as the sun crept through the blanket's holes and watched.

The sun's bright rays intensified and shined on the curled face of a woman

The floor was covered in boughs, and she slept deep. Half-asleep she lay, drifting back to her cabin at Wysox Creek's mouth in her memories. All seemed to be well for a brief moment. Slowly, she extended her arm across the imaginary feather bed to touch Sebastian. Sebastian, the sun shines! We must rise, we have chores to do. Her hand was cold and rough, breaking her dreams. She reached out to grab her husband's firm hand, but she was afraid to open her eyes. She thought in stupor, "No, it can't," she said. No! Finally, her hand grasped something that was twice the width of her husband's forearm. But it felt cold! It felt dead!

She stared at the horrors of captivity and opened her eyes again.

She held a pine branch in her hands. It fell to the ground like an iron rod. She ran back and forth from the light, seeking refuge in a dark corner. From the outside, sounds began to enter the hut. Her thoughts were invaded by the monotonous sound of a pestle crushing corn in a hollow wooden shaft. The air was filled with strange, guttural sounds that sounded like a foreign language. Her fear was heightened by the howl of Indian dogs. No! It cannot be!

"Ma?" A voice calls from outside the hut. "You alright in

there?"

She was able to hear her child's familiar voice and brought her back into reality. They are the children! They need to be monitored. Despite being held captive for so many months, they still didn't understand. It was their innocence that prevented them from understanding. She must take care of them! Sebastian wouldn't forgive her if they were to suffer any evil. Oh, Father! She muttered to herself, searching under the pine boughs in search of the last treasure. She felt the leather binding the pages in her hands. She held the large bible close to her chest. Your father had saved you from the fires that the savages had set you on to save the family's lives. This family bible must not be lost. It must be protected. It is your strength! Rise! With resolve and faith, face the day with all its horrors and it will pass. It will! Have faith!

She carefully slipped the bible under the boughs and ran her fingers.

Through her messy hair. She tied her hair back with an old piece of cloth and walked through the door to the ragged blanket.

To the wide-eyed children who were watching her, she said "Morning boys"

From around their small fire. Her eyes wandered all over the camp. She sat at the top of the hut, looking down at the river. One child was missing! She called Jane. "Jane!"

She listened intently, standing still. She waited, listening. "Boys! She asked, "Where's your sister?".
The three boys looked at each other curiously as they struggled with their shoulders.

another. The elder of the three said, "Don't Know," finally.

She said, "Oh, she will be the death for me yet!" She took a few.

She took a few cautious steps forward, shielding her eyes from rising sun. She looked around the village, looking for her daughter, but she couldn't find it.

One of the boys, kneeling down, said "She's just hungry Ma."

Poking at the fire using a stick. "We are all hungry."

"Well, you're just the man your Pa would like you to be.

She said "about fishing" to try to hide her panic.

The boy replied, "But Ma! They ain't biting anyhow!" "Ain't been in."

two days. The berries are almost finished." The boy looked curiously at the bustling Indian village. There were dozens upon dozens of corn racks that lit up in the sun. Numerous cattle grazed on the area to the west of the village. He asked, "Why don't they share with me Ma?" They've got lots. They always shared with you and Pa when they visited." He glanced at an old Indian walking slowly by their hut. "Why is Old Nicholas there? He was a good friend and shared a lot of our food at our cabin. We are in such a bad place, why doesn't he come with us?

She said, "War makes enemies of your friends." It's just how it is. Just mind your place, or you'll get the switch that your sister wants! I advised her to avoid the village. This applies to all of you!

"Yes, Ma," said the younger boy. "Would you like us to fetch?"

her?"

She said, "No!" "I want to tell you that I want you to go fishin' like I told you!" If you're looking for something to eat today, get on it!

"Yes, Ma," all three of them answered at once. One of them

Slowly, they picked up a line by the fire and the three of them trudged along the riverbank to the hut.

She called behind them, "And you mind Indians!" "And you

Avoid the blue-eyed ones too. They're just as mean and maybe even more!

"Hear Henry, Isaac, John?"

"Yes, Ma," climbed up the riverbank.

She grated her teeth as she walked slowly towards the village.

Trying to be as discreet as possible. She avoided eye contact and bowed her head to avoid offending any Indians. She was ignored by most. A few elderly women waved a wooden knife at her from the pots that they tend by their fires. But to her relief, none of them threw anything at her. Maybe it was the early hours. She noticed that none of the men seemed to be energetic in the morning. Most men prefer to sleep in their huts until noon, unless there was a festival, hunting, war party, or other reason. She thought it was a life without worries. They lived each day with little concern for the future, apart from the women. They worked in the fields and prepared for winter by planting the crops and hoeing the corn. They were the core of their society, just like their western counterparts. There was little to no change in the overall situation, but Indian women had far more control over the affairs of their society than white women.

> She moved around in the morning light, but she remained true to her original purpose.

shadows. She glided through the shadows of Ester's large cabin. It was silent.

> She let out a sigh, relieved that the Indian Queen had betrayed her.

She felt the most hate. After returning from the Battle of Wyoming, Ester proudly displayed the ring of scalps she had made. She heard Ester boast about lifting hairs of friends she used to call her friend. She saw the dark side of a savage's soul. It was something she would never forget.

> The dog ran up to her and sniffed her leg. The dog yipped and began

To howl. She ran from the castle immediately, not wanting to disturb the arrogant queen. With a gasp she stopped at the corner, staring at her daughter, who was standing by an Indian fire in rags and had one finger playing around her bottom lip.

She sat and watched as two Indians stood by the fire. One was a leather-clad Indian.

An old, wrinkled man stood with his skin tanned and wrinkled as he pounded a large wooden pestle into a stump. The little girl of white noticed that corn was spilling over the stump from time to time. It was captivating and she stood there, waiting for the right moment to grab some kernels.

Her mother noticed her staring and spotted the elderly woman by the

Fire also. The Indian woman looked at the white woman and child nervously, and let the wooden spoon that she was holding fall into the iron kettle she was tending. The white woman seemed to be daring her to get up. She wiped her hands on the buckskin dress and rose. Nonchalantly, she picked up a long twig.

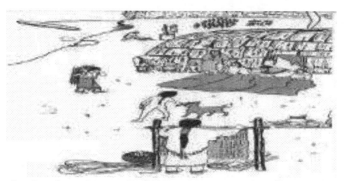

Slowly, the white woman backed away and bows her head. She rushed forward in a split second, picking up the child and turning her back to protect her from the old woman.

The switch of the old woman snapped immediately, and she fell heavily.

She landed on her back. She ignored the pain, and moved her child along, flexing both her arms to stop the blows.

The old man let out a laugh. He pulled a long braid onto his head.

He leaned his head back and watched the flight unfold before him with a sense of glee. The old woman's voice was harsh and he pressed the pestle once more. The pestle soon began to hum again.

The white woman was stopped beating by the old woman and turned to point.

The old man was frightened by the flashing switch. Before she could turn around, the child and white woman gained over 100 yards on her. She quickly spoke fast and threw her switch in the air at them. She finished her rant and returned to her pot as though nothing had ever happened.

Lydia Strope didn't stop until she reached their sanctuary

Little hut. She stopped at the fire and pushed the child out from under her. She rubbed her face against the welts and groaned from the pain. She said to her child, "I told you not to go to the Injuns!".

Jane innocently placed her finger in her mouth and said, "But I hunger!"

so, Mother."

Lydia bent her arm to ease the pain.

Looking down at the child in a state of shock. She said, "Oh, it's all good.".

Jane asked, "Ya mean that I ain't getting the switch?".

Lydia replied, "No," "I think there's been enough switching' for this."

she was going to die." "See what it will get you if you mess with the Injuns?" Imagine what the old witch would think if she had taken some of that corn.

Jane sat down beside an empty glass and said "I'm sorry Mother."

Clay pot by the fire. It was beautiful. She thought, "When is it going to end?" When is Papa going to come and fetch us from here? He went to fetch the soldiers and got us so long ago. She cried, "Where are they?".
"I fear the Indians and Tories have all the soldiers for months."

Lydia said it, lifting Lydia in her arms.

Jane asked, "And Pa?".
Lydia, recalling the events, said "Well, they said that they had,"

Brave men teased her by bringing in every new hair, claiming it belonged to 'Boss Strope. She figured that none of her hair was her husband after careful examination.

She added, "But I don't place much stock in their words,".

Chapter Twenty-Eight

The early morning fog was broken by the sun's rays, which reflected off many rocks and glittered on the leaves. Glutton men slept in slumber under branches and around numerous sized rocks. Some people sat on the rocks with their heads down and their chests bowed. Some others sat directly on top of moss-covered rocks. Others sat on the wet and cold earth. They wrapped themselves in their overcoats and blankets as best they could and draped themselves accordingly.

They were all watched by one pair of half-opened eyes. Boss Strope

He pulled his blanket tight to his chest and leaned back against the tree's rough bark. His feet sank into the soggy, black soil. He thought of his last two moccasins and looked down at his torn moccasins. Five new pairs had been with him when he started the expedition. He tried to rub his toes on the moccasins' leather, swearing that he would wear them until his feet fell off. His heavy eyelids fell, only for loud gasps to force his eyes back open. There was no movement, except for a few men looking for better positions to continue their painful sleep.

He gazed through the white fog all around him. He looked around the camp at the white fog.

It was lit up by silhouettes of sentries that shone like shadows. He watched their slow, careful movements of heads. Their eyes were always scanning the perimeter. He found comfort in their constant vigilance and vowed to follow suit when it was his turn to guard. He was startled by a slight drop of rain on his nose. It had stopped raining, he realized and wiped it off. Only drops of the leaves from above fell on the camp. He thought this, as he squirmed in his wet clothes, was a good thing.

Finally, he found a comfortable position and stopped.

squirming. In a matter of seconds, he knew that the officers would arrive to get them ready for the march through the terrible wilderness. He didn't mind, as he had more reasons to win Ester's village-his loved ones.

He sat back, following the leaf that danced on a gentle breeze.

Above his head. He drifted to his Wysox Creek homestead in his mind's eye. These quiet moments before dawn were what he loved. He would often rise early to walk down to the river and take a stroll before others. He would sit there and watch the waters swirling around him, as well as the slowly rising life. A fish would leap, leaving behind only an expanding circle and a splash. A blue heron could glide gently across the surface of the water. Hidden in a cove, ducks would flail their wings and quack. Sometimes, elk and deer would swim in the water. It brought him closer with God, thus closer to the things that really mattered.

The sound of an axe will often echo in the early morning light.

day. John, his brother, always rose early and cut wood first. It brought him peace, he said. They never ran out of firewood, even with him there.

Then he would stretch out and rise from Indian grass, along with the others.

Bank and walk back to the cabin to find Lydia, who is already busy at the hearth making the day's victuals. In the early hours of the morning, her smile was always infectious. He was always welcomed by it and the thought of it now brought a warmth to his tired bones. "Oh, my dear Lydia. My dear children. He whispered, "Old Father Van Valkenburg Isaac, Hermonos and all," he said. "I pray that you all return safely. Amen."

It was a thought that made his eyes water. That late May evening

Last night, an Indian stayed over with them. He was overcome by their kindness and began to hint at an attack on Wyoming. They were only twenty miles away from Tioga Point, the launch point for the attach. He took his rifle with him and began to travel for Wyoming in search of help in evacuation and information about the invasion. Colonel Denison sent some scouts down to his family to help them. However, to their horror, they found only the ashes of their cabins, barns and outbuildings upon arrival. In a rush to leave, the scouts split up to chase down any following men. Three others joined him in returning to the battle. Three other men took the river but did not. He was astonished at their fate and worried that their hair would end up on an Indian buck's pole. He was horrified at his family's fate.

He was not the only one who slept with him. "I'se feels the feelings, I do," said a deep and husky voice in the air.

Rudolf Fox was staring at him, and he lowered his eyes. He said, "Mein Goot! Don't worry." "You know, the wildens took my twice, they's did at dat, der second time together with yours," he said. The small, stout Dutchman nodded his head and raised his eyebrows. He said, "Ester will see that they're well-tended, she will.".

Ester! Ester!

His mind. He could just wrap his arms around her neck. He had witnessed her riding triumphantly on a captured horse, with the back facing forwards, into the fort, displaying a ring still full of bloody scalps to Colonel Denison, mocking him, and all of Wyoming, after the surrender at the last battle. It was difficult for her to move on the horse because she was wearing so many of her captured petticoats. Her head was adorned with a stack of equally tall bonnets that were all facing her backwards. She seemed almost like a joke, a cruel joke, and the most cruel of all times. She gave up the war club on the Wyoming bloody rock, cracking many a captured patriot's heads, all his friends. She incited the Indians. She ruled all the way along the Susquehanna. It would have never happened if she had opposed it, even with all the charm and trinkets Indian Butler could offer.

Boss Strope stated, "The rain has stopped.".
Rudolf wouldn't allow him to change the subject. "We're all rebuilding."

When der war is over. Lydia, you, mein and all our children."

Boss looked up at the leaf. "If any hair is damaged on any of these," Boss said.

"They have their heads, or is on some buck's post. All hell and Brant cannot save Ester form my wrath!" he stated.

"Amen to it," a voice spoke from the crowd huddled around.

tree.

"And if this all doesn't satisfy me, I'm going back to."

Boss stated, "The Hudson among my own." "We have a way of settling the differences with the savages."

Rudolf exclaimed, "Mein Shoe", while raising his foot from the ferns. He

He wiggled his feet through the remnants of a once-fine shoe. "I don't know if it'll take another crossing."

Boss said "Relax" as he thought of his worn moccasins. "We're

Nearing the head, rain's stopped so the water will drop not like yesterday." He was overcome by the thought of having to negotiate the steep, anthill-like mountains and then end up crossing the creek half a dozen times more yesterday.

Captain Franklin, slowly rising from ferns, replied "Yes."

It is far away from the tree. His tall frame appeared to grow from the ground as if it were his own creation. He knelt down and emerged with a rifle almost as tall as he. "We're getting close." He leaned forward and took out a rifle that was almost as tall as him. "I can taste them. He said, "Everyone is to look smart today, for we might have some sport!" and then he walked towards a group gathered by a large boulder.

Someone said, "That man scares my sometimes," from around the

tree.

Boss stated, "That's great," which means he scares all the enemies.

more. This is the devil we need for this job."

The voice replied, "Oh, he is a devil. I'll vouch that." "A

devil indeed."

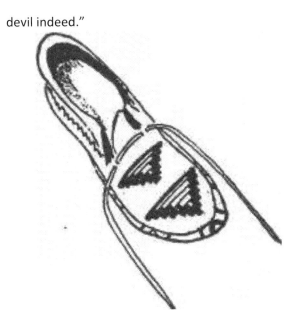

Chapter Twenty-Nine

The Indian village, nestled on the banks of Susquehanna, bustled with activity. Warriors shouted and screamed war howls. The air was filled with the sound of muzzles firing. All the Indians and their white Tory brethren gathered to the south Ester's village, watching intently the path.

Just below the water, canoes were seen plowing up the river.

Pine bough huts provided shelter for the village's captives. The braves ran to the huts and hurriedly landed the canoes. Some of them screamed loud war howls.

Lydia Strope leapt up from the floor in her hut. Tired

Their inability to get food and their desperate attempts to find any, drained her spirit but did not stop her curiosity. Her four children stared up at her with wide-eyed anticipation. They might have gotten a bite of food from this celebration.

Lydia lifted the ragged blanket door one sliver and aimed at the

village. She glancing over her shoulder, she stated, "Now, you kids, mind your places." "Don't draw attention to us. Just behave and think.

We'll all go out there to see what all the ruckus about is about." All four nodded.

She pulled the blanket aside and crawled out of the hut. The children were delighted.

She saw the crowd behind her. She reached out to protect her eyes from the bright sun and looked at the hooting Indians. She glanced back at her children, and moved them towards the village.

From the trail that led into the village, several shots rang out in the air.

Then came more exhilarating hoots, and calls. They were answered by an equally exhilarating series of hoots, yelps, and more. Queen Ester appeared suddenly at the castle's edge, her royal eye focusing down on the spectacle.

Five painted braves, all covered in black from head to feet.

Vermillion paint, strided from the trail to a clearing on south side of village, their fierce eyes looking straight ahead. A terrified white man struggled between them, tied to a leather strap. He turned his head to scan the faces around him and searched for any sympathy eyes. He was only able to see a white, elderly woman with four children who was emaciated standing at his side as he gazed back. His soul was not soothed by her concern and dreadful expression.

He raised his voice and twisted his head against a leather strap.

Over the clatter. "I am from Virginia!" I don't have a problem with the Northern people! "Why do you do that?"

One of the scattered white men in green coats was one of these.

The terrified man stepped beside him, as he was wearing a shirt he had just bought from a local shop. He said, smiling straight at the man, "A rebel is always a rebel, regardless of which colony he hails!" Now, be a sport! He laughed in a very sinister manner, adding "Don't ruin the fun!".

The gloating Tory was pushed aside by a brave man who stepped full in.

The prisoner's face. He made his face as distorted as possible, snapping his teeth. He suddenly locked eyes with the man, his bulging eyeballs darting about his head. Slowly, he turned one eye toward the castle of Queen Elizabeth II. He was followed by all eyes, even the prisoner's.

Her form tall and commanding, the Queen raised her head

high. The terrified, ragged white man was far away. She looked at her and slowly dropped her heavy eyes to ground. Slowly, she raised her hand and dropped it. She turned and disappeared into her cabin door.

Instantaneous chaos broke out among the Indians. Indifference by the Queen meant sport. From children to seniors, all ages, men and women, made a parallel line. They used war clubs, tomahawks and clubs in the space between. In a frenetic rush of anticipation, several brave men leapt in rapid jumps. The air was filled with yelps and war howls. To get a front row seat at the action, the Tories hooted and raised their hands. The white captive woman walked slowly up to the line but kept her distance. She held onto her children with both her hands and did not let them slip from her grasp.

The Virginian looked down at the line in front of him, cocking both his heads

He brushed his hair back, avoiding the matted and unmanaged hair that fell onto his face. He gasped, "What mischief?" He was answered by a chorus of whoops. "I'm just a farmer!" This is not something I did! Oh my dear God!

Oh, my sweet wife and children! Will she become a widow one day?

One of the Tories said, "You'll soon get your warrant served in its entirety!"

The screams soared above the wails. "You Rebel scum!"

Lydia Strope watched Lydia as she endured many of the tortures.

Tioga was in shock and awe. She couldn't seem to get away from the horrible rituals for some reason. It was all she could think of and she looked down at her children, wanting them to be safe from it, but not knowing that they would have to endure the terrible screams and bedlam. It was just the way of Indians. The terrified man stared at her with blank eyes. His eyes were a hint of tears, he looked back. She saw her husband in his eyes. She saw all American husbands on the frontier in his eyes.

The man was sent spiraling by a gruff push and kick from the behind.

Over foot into the slot between two lines. A war club smashed against his skull before he took his first step, twisting his head in an unusual motion. He fell instantly, moaning pitifully. He moaned for his mother. He moaned for his mother, the one from which all men descend. He longed for mercy or pity, but only whips and war clubs, tomahawks fists, sticks, and war clubs were able to answer his pleas. His face was covered in blood, and he pleaded for his life. His head turned in an odd motion. His neck seemed to be holding his head up, but his neck was only a thread. His bones cracked. He fell one, two, and three more times against the relentless blows and onslaught, before falling in a heap to the ground.

The Indians cheered and shouted. The Indian line closed in.

They circled around the corpse, relentlessly attacking it. After they had bludgeoned and shredded the corpse, both men and women ripped them apart to make room for their turn. The process continued until everyone had stabbed, spit upon, or kicked the corpse. The brave finally emerged from the crowd, placing the corpse on the ground with a trophy of blood in his hands. He shouted and held the Virginian's head high in the air, before spitting on the corpse once more. All of them left the scene of horror and congratulated each other, patting each others on the back.

Lydia struggled to keep the food in her stomach down

From the horrifying and bloody scene before her. She let go of the children and raised her hands to her cheeks. Jane ran towards the hut. The macabre sight captivated the boys as they stared ahead. She staggered towards the lump of flesh that was just a few beats ago a human being. Some bits of matted hair were scattered around the blood-soaked corpse. Unnaturally wrapped around the flesh were twisted arms and legs. The flesh was a purplish, human-like mass. It was alive with the horror and shock of her last sight. Through the mass of flesh, there was no sign of her other eye. She thought of pure hatred, and anger. She saw Ester, tall, regal and shining with bright eyes, condemning all acts of cruelty against the men who had been taken along with her and her children. They should be taken immediately to Fort Niagara, as she had demanded. They were held captive in cruel fetters, but they stumbled up the trail, led by one her most steadfast warriors, to see the unscrupulous Tories escorting the men to Fort Niagara.

> She gasped and lowered her hands. She looked around and counted.

Three children and not four. She ran to the boys, felt them all, and hugged them as she searched the area for her daughter. She remained focused on the corner of Ester's castle.

> Jane stood still and stared up at the dark-haired woman.

From head to foot, she was covered in silver trinkets as well as little brass bells. The woman smiled wide. Her hand reached out to the child.

> Jane smiled, and took a few cautious steps forward.

A firm hand from behind stops the motion.

Lydia pulled Lydia close to the child, and she stared defiantly at her Indian Queen. To protect her child from the dark apparitions before her, she buried her face in her chest and cuddled her close.

Ester looked at her with an understanding look, appearing to be looking back at her

You could sense the mother's desire to protect her child. She thought of her son, who was killed by the Yankees right before the Battle of Wyoming. She understood. She felt it. She couldn't condemn or admonish the mother's love for her children and their desire to protect them, no matter how unwise. She smiled and scratched her forehead before turning around and walking off.

Lydia held the child tightly and said "Oh Jane!" They both watched the Queen leave, and Lydia held onto the child tightly. Child, your father's flesh could stain her hands!

Jane stared down at the ground and said "No Momma." "Not Ester,

Remember, she and Pa are friends. She would not let anyone hurt him or us. Mama, you can see!

Lydia gently pulled the child away from her arms and gazed at them.

She was shocked. Sometimes, the innocence of the child shines through the hatred of times. She smiled and pulled the child closer. She hugged the child and rested her cheek on her shoulder. "Perhaps so," she said.

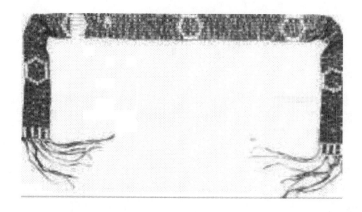

Chapter Thirty

Ira Stephens moved slowly through the underbrush, his rifle at his side. He moved slowly and let each branch that was grabbing at his clothes snap back in silence. He could see that his fellow scouts were doing the same. He looked down at his hands as he gripped his rifle. He imagined his fingers flicking the gun in an instant if the mysterious foe appeared before him. He heard Colonel Hartley's top command to "shoot on sight", despite their orders for stealth. The words echoed in his ears as he walked through the tangled hell.

> His relief was relieved when the underbrush grew and cleared ahead of him, giving him

Way to a grove full of trees high up on a high ridge. He gasped at the beauty of the grove, and the unspoiled expanse beyond it. These mountains offered such land, such beauty and such potential for wealth! It boggled his mind. He thought that this land could be a good place for a man after the war and all the hell. It was possible to create heaven where once hell dwelt. The thought was appealing to him, and he waited eagerly for the bright day that would come after the dark clouds of war receded.

One quick glance from a scout as he emerges from the underbrush to his

He noticed the side of his watch. Twelve others began to emerge behind him. They were spacing themselves in a wide, straight line to his left and right. They were stopped by Captain Franklin's waving hand.

Franklin raised his arm in the air until Franklin was at the end of the line

He nodded or waved to him. He raised two fingers in front of his eyes and motioned to the men beside him to move forward.

Stephens happened to be in Franklin's place. He looked over at Sergeant Baldwin, who was sitting on the opposite side of Franklin. Both men raised their rifles and walked silently towards the edge of the steep ridge after Franklin nodded.

Their attention was immediately captured by a slight whiff of curling smoke

attention. Baldwin looked over at Stephens with anxious eyes. He turned and made a swirling gesture to Captain Franklin. All along the ridge was the distinctive click sound of firelocks being cocked.

Franklin nodded in agreement of the clicks, and slowly crawled.

Moving forward, motioning to Stephens and Baldwin.

Franklin, Stephens and Baldwin drew closer to the edge.

They stare at it in fear, frightened of what lay before them. The smoke was coming from a hole in the bark hut's top, which is located in a small crook in the creek below. The men looked around at each other for any sign of movement. There was no movement, except for a woodpecker that began to climb a tree above the hut. The woodpecker's pecking began echoing throughout the grove, pounding the nerves of the restless people around it.

The men retreated from the edge of ridge. Franklin

He waved his right palm up and down towards the men, while pointing with his left to their eyes. Slowly, he moved slowly and pointed with his forked finger first to the right and then the left of the grove.

His alert eyes spotted him and immediately responded. Men spread

To surround the hut, move to the right and left.

Before he began crawling, he waited for the signal from the men on his flanks.

He moved forward once more. He suddenly stopped and pointed at his eyes, gesturing back to where he was pointing. He pointed at a man with wide eyes to his left.

The man nodded slowly and then turned around, quickly returning Colonel Hartley's message and alerting the horsemen.

Franklin let his hand drop to the tomahawk that was still in his belt.

He rubs it with the top of his long knife's handle. He stood, grasping his rifle with great care. The entire line of rangers moved slowly forward with a slow gesture of his arm. The rangers moved so naturally that the wood-pecker remained at his work, his pounding muffling any noises made by the rangers.

They were only a few feet away from Franklin's hut.

They were directed to stop. Every third man in line turned to face their enemy from the woods. The rest of rangers aimed their guns at the hut.

Stephens was left to cover their rears, so Franklin and Baldwin crept.

To the entrance of the hut. Franklin slowly eased his rifle towards the ground as he knelt at the entrance. He reached for his knife and tomahawk, then slipped them from his belt. Baldwin stood straight to his side and pointed his rifle at the door.

Franklin glanced at him briefly and then locked eyes with the door. He jumped through the blanket door and began rolling into the hut without warning. Baldwin followed his lead and began to fan his rifle around the inside of this door.

The door to the hut was watched by all the rangers, keeping their ears open.

Any signs of struggle in it were caught. Baldwin slowly stepped back and lowered his rifle. He looked around the grove in front of them and turned.

Franklin, holding his tomahawk, walked out of the front door.

He remained firmly in his belt, with his knife still in his sheath. He held a number of small hoops, his expression sour. The hoops contained a long, straight hair tied tightly by leather thongs around the middle of each hoop.

He dropped the empty hoops at their feet.

Rangers carefully examine the hair hoop. He winced as he turned the hoop over to its backside. He held them up and showed everyone the brightly colored backside. He said, "It's how they identify it for proper sales to those Crown fiends in Niagara!" "One color for one poor soul, and one for another." "What fiendish mind thought this? I don't know. If I find out and cross his evil paths, he'll die, I grant that!"

The woodpecker suddenly flung a swift wing from the grove.

One of the rangers asked, moving towards the hut. Franklin replied, "Yes." "But the fire's still hot and they left the

"They have trinkets to trade around," he raised the scalp hoop in disgust. "They cannot be far away, must have scattered just before we got here or been off on another hunt around." He extended his hand in a wide arc. "Be focused on finding them, but keep your distance. They'll be gone in a flash if they catch our attention. However, you should still keep an eye on them.

Everyone's eyes were pierced by a neigh at the top of the ridge. Captain Carberry sat on top of his mount, staring down at the hut. Franklin's footsore runner was also present.

Franklin called Franklin to the top of his list.

The ridge. "If you're quick, you might just catch one the rascals!"

Carberry gave a quick nod and waved his horses ahead. Hooves

The horsemen thudded across the top of the ridge and disappeared into the trees below. Anxious rangers followed the horsemen in a hurry, thirsty to take revenge on Captain Franklin's grisly trophy.

Franklin watched them disappear and bid them all fair hunting. He sat down and watched the last one disappear over the ridge, waiting for Colonel Hartley and all the ranks and file. His tired body began to feel dull and achy. He placed his scalp hoop in plain view so that everyone could see it as they approached.

He looked down in dismay and wiped his face against his own back.

He wore buckskin leggings in an attempt to remove the grime of death from them. But he feared that only the blood of the savages would be able to do so. He was certain that only after the savages had breathed their last, would the air be clean of their foul stench.

He pondered the idea and decided to make a vow.

Clear the air is best.

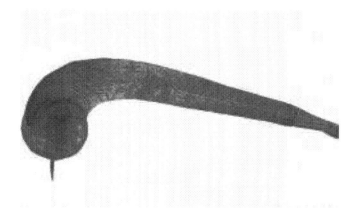

Chapter Thirty-One

Lydia Strope was overcome by the flames of her pine bough home. She reached for a half-shell gourd and took a sip of the contents. Jane was seated on Jane's lap and she offered her the gourd.

The child looked at his gourd, and he pushed it aside. He then began rolling him.

Her mother sat on her lap, and she flipped her head. Her mother was haunted by her empty eyes.

Lydia looked at the child and didn't say a word. No

Their hunger could be soothed by words, however. The empty gourd was placed on her lap and she began to brush her hair. They both jumped up as John, Henry, Isaac, and Henry trudged along the riverbank behind their hut. They noticed the empty hands of the boys and their spirits quickly dropped. The boys looked at each other and plopped down next to the fire.

John stated, "There's no fish bitin' no more Ma." "The berries

It's all dried up and I can find no wild plums nor potatoes anywhere."

Lydia replied, "I know my son," but don't worry none, you've done it."

You did everything you could. It will make yer pa proud, and all your boys, to hear it."

Henry looked down at the empty plate and asked: "What are we to eat?"

half-gourd shell. "More water?"

Lydia stated, "You can just wait and pray to the Lord." He'll see us

through this."

John stood and gazed up and down at the riverbank. He said, "Ain't right."

said. "I can understand why the Injuns don't share with us but not why other white people around don't. Provost has a lot of land up there. Secord's apple tree is just around the point, as well as Daniel Moore and his ferry. "Ain't they all got any heart?"

Lydia: "No, son. I don't believe that they have."

said. She noticed the anger in her son's eyes and decided to warn him against doing any reckless acts. Her back was still tender from her rescue of Jane from the wrathful old Indian witch who had attempted to steal a bite of food. "And don't let any of you go about your places!" It's impossible to predict what they would do if we gave them a fake call. Let them be as cruel as they are.

John replied, "But Ma," John said that they's got so many! It's not Christian.

Lydia replied, "No, it's not." "But all people don't follow the word."

They were alerted by a sudden noise in the village. They were shocked to discover that there was a sudden commotion in the village.

Eyes followed the Indians, Tories and others who clamored to the north of the village. Two men led a train full of pack-horses loaded with food and other necessities into the village.

John stated, "There's Secord now." "Looks like Secord has arrived to

Trade." He raised his hand to protect his eyes from the scorching sun. "I don't know the name of that man, I have never seen him before."

Lydia sat up and looked at the noise again. Any

Change, whether in person or otherwise, could be welcomed with some consideration and perhaps even pity by a starving Christian mother and her children. Jane sat down on her lap and stared at the train of pack-horses.

She said, "Now, all of you stay put!" She rubbed her scalp, adjusting her hair.

He walked towards the train. She called out to John, "make sure all the other people stay put!"

She sat down on the train and tried to be inconspicuous until she reached the platform.

Right now. She carefully walked around the whites trading with the sutler at Tioga Point. She was suddenly turned towards the sound by the sharp crackling of an ox whip.

An old man Secord was seen cracking the whip he had been given in trade. With each crack of the whip, a cruel smile appeared on his face. It seemed to be a fascination for him.

The other whites were not as enamored by his new toy and stepped instead

He preferred to trade with his partner, while admiring his latest acquisition.

Lydia saw her moment. Lydia carefully approached the whip.

Cracking man, he waited until he had finally tied the whip to his belt and looped it up before taking his last steps towards him. She lowered her head and stood in submission before him.

He shook his head and said "Why, if not Boss Strope's wife?" "You still about? Sometimes I question Ester's judgment. Boss is an Indian name for Bostonian. This is because they believe all the hubbub comes from Boston. They don't give rebel dogs the names they deserve! He should be punished for his treachery, along with his family!"

The others were attracted to his harsh words. They all

In anticipation of some sport, he turned to his loud voice and turned toward him. His trading partner viewed the unusual behavior with an attentive, but cautious eye.

Lydia bows again and says, "Yes sir." "Be that it may, I have

Children who are almost starving in this area." She looked at the flour bags on the backs of the pack-horses and thought, "This is a terrible place for children." "A little flour from your grace would certainly go a long ways in relieving their suffering."

Secord shouted, "What impudence do Rebels possess!" "Let them starve! You too! "Nits breed lice," he scoffed. "Where is your Congress now?" Your Denison is missing. Is that Zebulon Butler, a young upstart, and Hollenback, a penny-pinching Hollenback missing? Their warm hearts made them feel safe and healthy, no doubt! Be gone! "The sufferings of a damn Rebel are not my concern!"

Lydia said "But sir!" before collapsing on the ground and climbing up.

The man. He tugged at her buckskin britches and she cried, "My children shall..."

starve! Do you want to play with your conscience?

He gruffly kicked her aside, saying "War has no conscience!". She let tears run down her worn cheeks. She rose to her knees.

Through tears of anguish, I stare at the man.

He yanked the whip from his belt and said "You wretched shench!" He snarled in anger, only checking the swing when his partner intervened between him and his target.

"Stand clear, Cyrus! "Son or not, this lash shall swing!"

Cyrus screamed, "No father!" He knelt down and helped the father.

She helped a distraught woman get to her feet. "She is not to be blamed for her husband's rebellion!"

Secord snapped at his feet the whip. Secord jumped, his eyes flashing

In disbelief at the father.

Secord

He exclaimed, his eyes bulging in the back of his head. He extended his arm wide and was ready to whip his son and the woman.

Lydia shouted, "No!" "Are not you the man who once took?"

His place on the Committee of Safety at Wyoming Were you not once trusted with our lives and property? Did you not once be close friends with Nathan Denison and Mathias Hollenback, whom you now despise? You would make a woman and your children die from the failures of others. What happened to the once-good man?"

Through gritted teeth, Secord declared "War." "You Yankee rascals!"

He wouldn't let a man live in peace upriver, but insisted that he choose sides when he wanted neither." He paused and surveyed the eyes of those around him. "You took me to the Simsbury Mines, but for leveler heads."

Congress, I would still be there in hell! These acts were not my fault!

You impudent rats!"

Lydia shouted, "I had nothing else to do with that!".

Secord looked up at the whip with glaring eyes and said "Then it will be the innocent that pays for the sinsof the guilty." "But someone will pay!"

Cyrus called Lydia, twisting Lydia behind his back to protect her.

From the whip, "are your mad?"

He heard a strange, shrill voice behind him calling "Secord!" He

The Indian Queen stood tall and regal as she turned her head to see her. She reached out to touch the blanket of blue wrapped around her. The blanket shone underneath her rich, extravagant, and glitteringly embellished dress. In the quiet air, her moccasins and blue-colored skirt jingled like bells. She made a slow, steady step forward. She said, "No more!".

Secord gasped in frustration and lowered his whip. Secord rolled it

He leaned forward, gripping his hands tightly, and stomped off towards the Indian village cursing everyone behind him.

Ester stood still for a moment, and then looked at Lydia, who cocked her head.

head around Cyrus. She smiled at her and lowered her eyes before slowly walking off.

Lydia said behind her, "Thank you!".
Cyrus told the curious, "Do not worry," he said.

Indian Queen. Lydia smiled, wiping her tears-strewn eyes.

Cyrus waited for the Tories to melt away in their cabins before he did so.

Before he led Lydia behind a pack horse, He reached for a small bag with flour and motioned to Lydia to put it in her dress' ragged folds.

Lydia's grateful eyes were beaming back at him.

Cyrus stated, "Take this flour to good use." "This war makes mad!"

Men of once-sane men. It will soon pass, so everything shall be as it was." He glanced down at the woman asking him questions. "It may never be the same. But I will not let a woman's or her children's death on my conscience when this madness ends. Be quiet about the flour. I will try to sneak more from Father's shops at night. They will be canoed down by me. We have to be careful as fathers account for every ounce of food and every shilling. But we will manage. I will think of some trivial excuse or other such thing."

Lydia exclaimed, "Oh, God has sent his angel." The tears poured.

down her cheeks again.

He said, waving to the woman to go: "There are no angels at war."

Her hut. "Only demons can enjoy its hell."

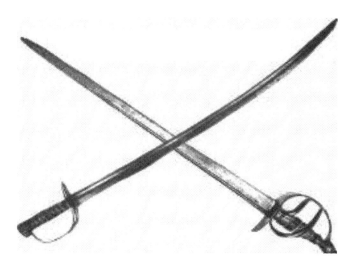

Chapter Thirty-Two

Colonel Hartley slowly approached the ranger, sitting cross-legged before a single bark hut. He looked around the hut, then turned his attention to Franklin, his eyes following his gaze towards the object of his seething anguish.

>Franklin stated, "Who knows to which poor soul this hair belonged?"

He turned his attention to the pile of empty hoops and pushed them aside with his hand, shifting his gaze. He took a few and tossed them in the air, disdainfully. He said, "And who knows which hair was meant to be these?" and he flung one of them in the air with his free hand. "Perhaps yours! "Perhaps mine!" He glanced beyond the colonel at the sea of eyes straining for his attention. He added, "Perhaps all of them!".

>Hartley stated, "Yes, but they won't be used for good purposes."

He bent down to grab one of the hoops. He threw it in the stream, which was only a few yards from them.

>The bark hut was shaken by a shaking sound.

eyes to it.

>Robert Covenhoven, a leader of a group of afirmatives, said "Made strong."

Half a dozen other Scouts were also present, with all sharing the same disgusting look. He added that the Scouts were made to last the next season, and he circled the hut before coming to a halt in front Franklin. He noticed the scalp and said "Probably a Yank's hair." "Matted so."

Franklin rose immediately and stood tall and straight in front of the Pennamite Scout. Even though Covenhoven was taller than average, his tall frame dwarfed Franklin. He grinned through his teeth, "Matted! Eh, that makes sure a damn Pennamites haircut!".

Covenhoven stood firm, slowly shaking off his head and tonguing.

He smuggled a piece of tobacco in his cheek. He tilted his head and spit a large amount of tobacco juice onto the ground.

Franklin lost his hand with his tomahawk.

Covenhoven raised his gun ever so slightly, and he spat again.

This time, Franklin is closer.

Hartley stated, "Now see here gentlemen," he said, "one at a time!"

He added, putting himself directly in front of the men. He saw all the eyes looking at him, Yankee as well as Pennamite. He knew that this was a time when a leader should unite and solve the conflicts in his command that were threatening its cohesion. He rubbed his chin and raised his hands to separate the men further. He said, before the men could protest, "We," "all of us," and they were separated even further. We have very few chances to win laurels. But it is what it is! We are facing a most dangerous and vile foe! They are strange and vigilant as they avoid danger when they are among us." He looked around slowly. They fight bravely when they are within their country. We aren't just close, we are in their country! We must not allow past disagreements to divide us, but instead unite against this potentially deadly foe. It should give us joy to think that our country is being served and that we fight for the defenseless and innocent!" He raised both his arms and answered him with a series of huzzas. He stood firm and surveyed both men.

Covenhoven was first to move, slowly lowering the rifle to offer his.

Hand to the Wyoming Scout, a small, but sincere smile creeping across him face.

Franklin's stern expression gave way to a smile.

Both men laughed and walked towards the pack-horses.

Doubt in search of whiskey barrels.

Hartley directed a few soldiers to mingle around him to "dismantle that vile structure".

One of them asked, "Put that to the torch sir?".

"No, no, by Gods, would you like to announce our advance towards the

entire Six Nations?" he quipped.

The man replied, "No sir,".

Hartley stated, "Then be all about it man", taking a few steps towards

some officers approaching him.

Captain Spalding stated, "They were some mighty fine phrases," and "mighty fine, indeed they were."

Hartley looked at the other Wyoming officers and Pennsylvania officers, "And I meant each syllable." "One enemy at the time!"

He raised his eyebrows and a few shaking heads replied.

They glare at one another. Some of them nod.

Sweeney asked, gazing up at the dimming light in the treetops.

His words were answered by the thunder of some hooves. Captain Carberry stepped in front of them, along with half a dozen Light Horses. He looked down and shook his head in dismay. "Sir! He reported that he didn't see any devils' hair or hide.

Hartley stated, "You can make your tent here, Mr. Sweeney.". "Ensure that the men get enough rest, for we may have sport tomorrow."

Sweeney replied, "Yes sir", already waving his arms, and motioning

For the men to set-up camp.

Hartley is called "Lieutenant King" by Coven-hoven

retreating scouts. He stopped, turned and leaned on his rifle. Through his tired eyes, he looked back at the colonel. The colonel could not speak, but he was content to have his words.

Hartley quickly stepped over to the man. Hartley nodded his head.

I gave the man a thorough inspection, noting his ragged and torn clothes. Some spots of red were visible in his worn clothes.

Hartley thought about his sore knees after he had to bend down.

He crawled on his hands, knees and feet over the difficult trails. He was reminded of his own struggles in wading through ooze, mire and mud. He traveled the trail, but he was shaken to think about the hardships that scouts like this brave soul had to endure on the flanks.

King finally replied, "Yes sir.".
Hartley replied, "Yes," Hartley added, "on the morrow will we set out all of the

earlier. It is likely that we will have our first encounter with our wily enemies. I would like you to join Captain Franklin's advance party with Captains Boone, Brady, Peter Grove and Covenhoven. You will travel light and fast to Sheshequin.

King turned to the pack-horses. Captain Franklin was already there

Covenhoven and other returning men from the party gathered around a barrel whiskey and enjoyed it. King replied, "I see no problem at all with that sir." He lowered his hand from the rifle and wiggled his dirty bag around. The colonel opened the bag and found it empty. "There is plenty of boiled beef, but there aren't enough ash cakes. "Seeing' how we don't have time for fires, I bet my bag isn't the only one in this lot."

Hartley replied, "Yes," Hartley stated. Hartley said, "Yes,"

Night, but we have to make them low enough that each man can eat and carry his own food for the next day's march. Only use the hardest wood and heat the stones for cooking, then put out the fires.

King nodded. King nodded.

He pounded the scout on his back. "I've

I heard about your troubles with family and friends, as well as your encounter with the savages before we marched. Your escape was amazing and I am grateful for it. We will see to it that this nonsense is stopped, or at the very least we are as troubled by our foe. We will show the Six Nations that we can deliver a punch as well as take one.

King rubbed his rifle stock, saying, "Oh, King, I have trouble for!"

They are right here, they are mine."

Hartley replied, "Of that I'm certain." Hartley turned to see the scout off and he turned

The officer is still behind him.

Stoddert stated, "I heard what your said to the Scout sir." "Fire for

all?"

"Yes, but we don't want to make public our decision.

"Presence for all to see."

Stoddert replied, "Very well sir," and turned smartly away to "the men's."

stomachs shall thank you."

Hartley was preceded by another officer who could sit on a

Nearby boulder Sweeney replied, "The stores sir." "Already three pack horses are empty of their loads. Two of them carried whiskey and one flour." He looked around at men sitting around fires, and began to drink from their canteens. Hartley was his only hope.

Hartley stated, "Look at where we are." Hartley said, "Look at what we are already doing."

They have to endure. It's hard enough to endure it all on an empty stomach. I don't think so. On this miserable march, not a single word has been spoken of discontent. I don't intend to make them grumble. Let them eat, and have fun, because it could be their last night on earth. We are also in the middle of the enemy's territory. Sweeney eats, too, and he plunders Wyoming and the West Branch! This night, everyone will eat and drink their fill. We will replenish our stores with captured items."

Sweeney wouldn't have it. Sweeney would not have it.

He said, "Starting a revolution?".
Hartley asked Hartley straight: "Have ye never seen General Knox?"

faced. He raised an eyebrow and moved about his waist to try to get a response.

Sweeney tried unsuccessfully to keep his smile from corroding his stern.

look. He thought of the colonel who sat on top of a boulder in the middle the unmanaged wilderness, his one leg resting under an arm, while the other dangles free over the boulder's edge, and he was drinking copiously from a canteen of whiskey. Sweeney stated, "I have seen General Knox.".
"And I heard Colonel Glover's remarks about the man."

Hartley said, with a wide grin that stretches from ear to ear, "Well, there it is," to ear across his round little face. "Oh, Captain Sweeney, let them eat and be merry, for their spirit demands it, especially in this dismal place. The thread of leadership is never so thin than when faced with troubles and predicaments such as these. So drink and be merry as one can on this God-forsaken march through this God-forsaken wilderness! Remember, in the

end, it is for liberty we march!"

Chapter Thirty-Three

All along the valley, the hollow sound of water drums could be heard. Ester's Town was illuminated by great fires at dusk. Dogs howled and wanted to be part of the war songs and chants that resounding through the air. The warriors danced in their full war costume, with gruesome swirls in red, black and white. Their feathered heads swung around a single pole. Eight hoops were hung from the pole, each one tucked with hair.

Musicians continue to pound the drums faster and harder.

Time and called out their war songs. The braves responded with applauding war whoops. The dancers danced with great care around the pole. They flashed their teeth and bulged their eyes when they heard the music. Their glowing eyes and painted skin gave them an incredibly terrifying look. Young women stood just beside the circling soldiers, shouting encouragement and cheerleading them on.

As she did every time, Lydia watched from her Queen Ester's hut. Standing now and again, her hands resting on her hips, she prayed silently in the face the heathen rite. The eight scalps she had taken at German Flats were a bragging Tory, which she heard. The eight deaths brought joy to the slayers, and sorrow to the families of the victims.

She shook her head in an effort to forget the terrible memories.

Observed during her time at Ester's town. She cannot count how many scalps she saw, and how many poor souls were left to die in the gauntlet. She saw the Indians create bales of scalps and each one was painted on the back with a specific color so that it could be identified. She was shaken by it all. The British Empire funded a human trade in scalps. This is a terrible trade!

Her heart stopped beating when the drums stopped.

She could hear the anticipation in her ears. She looked at the flickering light in search of any signs of trouble but nothing was certain. Ester's Palace was thronged by musicians, hooting braves and young women, who led the rest of them.

Lydia told her wide-eyed, sitting children "Stay put,"

Their humble fire pit. Their fear told her to stop repeating herself. The children have been happier ever since Cyrus Secord delivered a steady supply flour. She thought that a full stomach seduces all.

Ester's tall form was visible as she leaned forward to view her.

The Tories in green stood out above the rest, as did the Tories. The smart-looking tri-cornered hat he wore with a cockade, cocked to one side, was defiantly positioned beside her. He seemed hesitant to give any authority to her. He appeared to be a prince in his own eyes.

Ester raised her arms and revealed her brightly-adorned clothes

underneath her blanket. The reflecting firelight reflected off her huge necklace of white with a cross attached. Instantly, everyone fell silent. Her hand pointed towards her palace's door. The door was half open when a man emerged slowly, pulling his hunting shirt down. He lowered his head and walked towards the gathering, keeping his head down.

Ester spoke in her native language loudly before referring to the

advancing white man.

Lydia noticed the man's cocksure stride, which Lydia knew because they had all been there.

It, the Pawlings and the Wintermoots and Van Gorders. And this traitor, Van Alstyne. With a sharp stare, she glared at Van Alstyne with an indifferent look, trying to get his attention for just a moment to express her disgust over him and his like. All the hatred of a traitor would be evident in her eyes in a blink of an eye. The man, full of self-importance, ignored her and stood tall in front all.

"I've been in great peril at the Wild Yankees in Wyoming!"

He said it, pausing to add effect. "There, I pretended friendship only for their designs to be discovered! They are now mine! They marched from Fort Muncy three days ago, almost seven hundred strong. "Maybe many more!" A whisper echoed through the crowd.

"And now they will know we are aware of them!" The man in the

Van Alstyne was astonished by his fine tri-cornered hat. He pulled and played with a pair fine gloves in his hand, raising them in contempt. He said, "They will figure out where you have gone.".

Van Alstyne wouldn't be outstripped. "They don't know where I am."

He said, "I have gone." "For all they know, I have gone on wind!"

The man laughed. "A north wind, straight towards Tioga!" Rebel Butler and Denison know what you are all about. They are able to see what you are thinking and have no doubt guessed your intentions."

Van Alstyne asked, "Why Captain Butler sir? He leads?"

Hartley and the Rebels!

The Indians heard a gasp and then a hush. The white men

They looked around at the crowd of painted and shocked faces, wondering what had happened to their white neighbors.

Walter Butler did not wonder. He knew exactly what was wrong and he knew it well

them. The Yankees made a solemn promise to them that they would not participate in this fight, particularly their leaders. He said, "See!" He said, "See how the Yankee speaks using a forked tongue?" He cradled his thumbs in the large belt of black around his waist and waited for the murmurs that would die. We must be ready to meet the lying Yankees!" They will feel our full wrath this time! My father's misplaced mercy will not be found within his son's heart! "In my heart!" He thumped on his chest, the gloves in his hands. He added, "I have suffered too much in their prison at Albany!" His eyes filled with deep pain as he reflected on the scene. He closed his eyes, lowering his head to the chest and slowly dropping his entire hand of gloves to the thigh. It was as if he was overcome by grief and purpose. A few fellow Tories quickly translated his words into their native languages. His declaration was followed by war whoops, cheers and huzzas.

Butler waited for the full impact of his act, keeping his head down.

be communicated to him by words. His eyes were rolling around in corners, half-closed, as if he was trying to trick them. The crowd soon became a frenzy to his delight, but the Indian Queen's haughty voice stopped them. She raised her arms and mumbled something in her native language. She slowly dropped her hand into her blanket and exposed a tomahawk, as all eyes were watching. She raised the tomahawk high above her head and yelled her terror.

Pandemonium reigned. Pandemonium reigned.

They took oaths to each other, swearing that Yankee Denison would be held responsible for his broken promise by paying with their lives! All Rebels would be punished with their lives. Their bravery would endanger their lives. To spread the news about the bold Yankees', Rebels' advances into their country, Queen Elizabeth and other chiefs sent runners in all directions.

The Tories were formed around their well-dressed captain. Raising

He raised his head in triumph and shouted orders to the other one. He finally got on his horse and announced that he would be carrying the word to Chemung, Kanadasaga. He would then mount a counterstrike to the Rebels, all the way to Wyoming. He left, ranting about how it would take another week to get such a large group of men, encumbered with such a massive supply train, to reach Tioga. They would then be ready to strike the Rebels until their hearts were full of blood forever.

Ester and the Indians ignored the white boastful man. Ester declared that they would do whatever they could, regardless of whether the white men bragging about their abilities were present.

Everyone's attention was diverted from Ester by a screech coming from a scalppole. The pole was pounded mercilessly by a large chief who urged others to join him in a strike to stop the invading troops. It didn't take long for it to respond. The braves scattered, quickly gathering their weapons and other accoutrements in preparation for the fiery war. The chief quickly led a large party of ninety braves along the southern approach to the village. Their heart-tingling wails faded in the distance beneath the pale moonlight.

Lydia slowly moved away from the growing chaos, finding her way

Through the shadows, she returned to her refuge by the riverbank. She eased into her dark bark hut, content to see her children's faces staring up at her.

One of them asked, "What's the matter Ma?".
She said, "Your Pa's Coming," with her first smile to stretch.

In months, her face has changed dramatically. Thank God, your Pa is finally coming with the soldiers!

Chapter Thirty-Four

The advance party hovered around four trees that looked curious, and stripped their bark from their trunks. They stood one after the other along the trail. Their trunks were covered in red-painted symbols and figures. Figures that have arrows running through them. The hands of their enemies painted headless figures.

One of them finally asked, "What's the deal?".
Another called, "Pay it no attention." "The rest is fast!"

We must keep moving forward, we are approaching!

Despite his pleas, no one came forward. They sat still, all

Looking at the figures, and the dark woods ahead, Many of them anxiously checked the primes in their flash pans. They sat silently, pondering their situation.

One of them said "These", stepping forward and pointing.

At the signs in the early morning sunlight, "show how many scalps were taken, of men in armour." He pushed his rifle barrel towards the set of figures opposite him. "These are not in arms. He drew his tomahawk out of his belt and tapped into the marks. "These are their losses. I intend to increase them until they can find a tree large enough to paint all of it onto it!" He pulled his tomahawk out of the tree and walked to a sapling, its top bent and wrapped around its trunk. He said, "This is a sign they are strong and together."

Hacking the sapling. "But not for too long, if you can help it!" A man asked.

"That's Jenkins," one answered another. "The one taken in by the Injuns

Put in the hole at Fort Niagara. He knows them well. He is all they fear, and they are."

Jenkins stated, "For good reasons," and began hacking away at the rest.

images. He finally contained his anger and took a deep, exhaling breath to regain his composure. He raised his rifle and pointed down the path. "Let's give them more to draw their ridiculous pictures about, shall?

He was followed by all of them, each with a rifle at his side. Their speed and determination increased due to the boastful signs posted on the trees. They soon began to glide down the path silently, with their woodsmen watching them closely. They trotted through ravines and hollows, eager to vent their anger. Many of them noticed a huge outcropping made of rocks that jut from the deep green veil of tall and high-heeled cedars. This slowed their pace slightly. Franklin, Covenhoven and Jenkins slowed down and raised a hand in an effort to stop them. They paid no attention to the sight but to the tingling sensation around their necks.

Franklin: "We're getting close, but I think there are twenty miles."

said. "We should slow down and wait for the column."

Jenkins and Covenhoven nodded, returning to the men.

They began to spill from the trail. They smiled at each other, forgetting their tingling necks. Their eyes widened with terror at the sight beyond them, causing a tingling sensation in their necks. They instinctively turned around when they saw the rifles of all the men.

The trail was dominated by a group of men in painted shirts, who stood at attention. Men

They were also surrounded by others, and the two sides came upon each other so quickly. The white demons were being stared at by a huge, red-colored warrior who was wearing their lead. His eyes became more angry. He raised his gun.

Instantly, both parties fired at the same time. White smoke

The narrow path was obscured by clouds. Angrily whizzing balls flew through the air, crackling branches overhead and thudding into ground. The Indians erupted in a mad roar, but the whites held fast in the smoke and advanced with a yell towards a mass of bullet-ridden red-painted inert flesh along the trail.

A few sporadic shots were taken at the advancing aircraft.

The whites whooped. They ignored them and ran, their adrenaline fueled hunt taking over their emotions. They could not stop themselves from committing suicide.

Franklin and Covenhoven both ran in the direction of a crook hidden in a tree

Each person fumbled with their powder horns as they tried to make a run at the red men. Franklin reached Covenhoven half a step ahead, and slipped his weapon into the pocket to stabilize his shot. Covenhoven was not discouraged and he threw his weapon to the ground. Both shot simultaneously, and Covenhoven twirled a brave along the path. The brave rose quickly, running wild from the angry white devils' hornet's nest.

"Get up! Franklin called him behind. "Lay fire."

Insist on them before they disappear into the forest!

Many men ran up and fired blindly along the trail, but to no avail. Franklin said "It's okay," and took no notice of their shots.

But it can terrify wildlife nearby, sending them running for cover. "Ya put God's fear in 'em!" Nothing scares the Be-Jesus more than a ball flying behind them! They'll be able to see it. They won't be as anxious to fight the next time."

Covenhoven rose and fired once again down the trail. He exclaimed, "Rascals!"

said. "But I think I wonged one of them!"

Franklin laughed at Franklin's reference to the twirling brave. Franklin smiled at his reference to the twirling brave.

He said, "I did too, by God, so I do.".
Both laughed and ran back to the fallen heroes on the trail.

Jenkins exclaimed, rising from his bullet-ridden body. The chief's face was nothing but a reddish glob of flesh. A fresh red spot appeared atop his skull crown attesting to one of the men who proudly displayed his scalp.

Jenkins stated, "Can't tell him who he really is," "account for his face being all

Shot up. He's a chief Muncy, I think."

"Who the hell cares?" Moses Van Campen stated, "Just so he's gone is all that matters." He walked over to the man who was displaying his scalp and said, "Seeing how no one knows fer certain who dropped the painted devil ball, is anyone going to protest this man claiming his scalp?"

The men quickly reloaded and replied, "Hell no!"

and verify their weapons. "There are more places than that one came from anyway!"

Franklin said, "Fine shots for all," while bending down to examine.

The Indian's face. "But next time, spread your shots out more, lads. That way, you can do more damage.

Captain Carberry and his Light Horse galoped madly up the mountain path. He said, reining in his horse and bringing him to a halt in front of the man with a scalp.

Franklin stated, "Yes, I met a party equal in number and let them have it." "Got one for certain and won another. They've hightailed Tioga back, but they've sent one of the painted rascals to hell!" He raised his head and looked at the scouts. He asked, "No one's hit is it?".
"Hell no," came a quick reply. "Hell no!"

Covenhoven stated, "Then make sure your rifles are in good condition." "For that,

The hell you mentioned is right up the trail and eager to meet us. We have to make sure that we can fulfill their wishes! We will meet them and send them to hell!

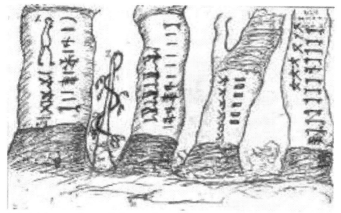

A sketch by eyewitness of pictographs carved into trees on Pennsylvania Indian Trails 1779.

Chapter Thirty-Five

Hartley leaned down and began to examine the corpse of the Indian chief. Hartley reached for the Indian's pouch and began to look through it. He threw the contents back on the ground after a while. He asked Captain Franklin, his side, "How was he provisioned?".

"He had plenty powder and ball, some corn cakes, and jerked meat.

Franklin looked down at the trophy knife in his belt and said, "I got a gourd to make a canteen." He added, "I got his knife belt." "The rest is split among us."

Hartley replied, "Very well." Hartley said, "So they were well provided for."

"War" means that they have come to our aid."

Franklin stood tall next to him and shook his head. "Oh, no sir," he

said. "They weren't coming to parley; they assured me of that!" They fired just as quickly as we did when they saw us!

Hartley: "Then, I take it that you both stumbled upon one another."

said.

Franklin rubbed his eyes and shook his head. "But who came?"

He asked, "Out the victor?" "We did."

Hartley said, rising slowly from his body, "They know of us for sure." "You say an equal number of savages has more or less met with you?"

"Yes sir," Franklin said. "Yes sir," Franklin said.

His surprise at his reaction made him reconsider. "Well, one of our team won one, don't know how many more balls hit their mark. You can see that most of them aimed at this rascal.

Hartley stated, "I see, and I do it with deadly marksmanship."

The unrecognizable face is the dead man. "Be that it may, now is the time to move quickly. The element of surprise is most certainly gone. Gentlemen, it's time to continue the long march! If we want to succeed, we must get to Tioga before they can gather their forces. Are you with me?

He was answered by a rousing chorus huzzas.

He said "Very well," and nodded his head in approval. He said, nodding his head in approval.

There will be one exception. Captain Carberry, you will continue with the advance scouts. We want prisoners, not scalps. We must learn as much as possible about the enemy's behavior!

The ranks and file formed immediately and marched up to the trail.

Scouts marched to the front, with horsemen taking over the flanks where possible. They marched one by one past their fallen foe. Some looked down at it with a bitter look, others ignored it and focused on what was ahead. Some obstinate people were able to slow down enough to give the body a quick kick or poke it using their bayoneted or rifled muskets. One or two even tried to spit on it.

The men in the column moved effortlessly down the more level terrain.

This valley is compared to the difficult path that runs along Lycoming Creek. Each of their exhausted steps were fueled by anticipation of a promised battle that would fuel them beyond what ordinary men can endure.

Hartley believed that sometimes quality is more important than quantity.

The spirited woodsmen trundle along the trail, mile after mile. They inspired the regiment's regulars. He was impressed by the behavior of all and felt proud to have witnessed their resolve. An immediate alarm was raised when he noticed a sudden slowing of his steps. He quickly strode towards the column's front, passing nervous eyes as he went.

He called out to a horseman, who was retraining his horse in front of him.

him. "What?" He approached the horse, putting his hands on its flanks and looking up at the trail.

"The Scouts found a spot where they could anticipate the arrival of their troops.

The horseman reported that close to seventy warriors had been slept down in the previous night. It's an abandoned village with some corn hills and mounds around, but no structures.

Hartley nodded his head in agreement, "Very well," Hartley stated. "Then we

It is not worth the effort. Tell Captain Carberry and the Scouts to keep going, we must reach Tioga by the next night!" He pulled himself off the horse and admitted that the slight relief felt good for his sore and aching legs. He stiffened his back, grinning against the pain. He yelled to the column, "Push On!" It was now moving again in front of him. Push on, God bless you, keep pushing on!"

They were exhausted after a few more miles. Men spilled

From the ranks, only for them to rise quickly from a quick kick and prod by their sergeants or officer. Hartley watched the whole thing with his head down to his chest. He mumbled, "We must stop!" He noticed that no one was following his orders and he fell to the ground, shouting "halt!"

He didn't have to repeat the order.

In exhaustion, men sank to the trail's edge. Horses

They sighed in relief at the offer of their masters.

Hartley said, "We will rest here for a while and then we'll continue."

He lifted his tired body from the ground, muttering the order. He said, "The Light Horse men shall stand guard, half-on picket and half-at rest." And he let his exhausted body sink completely to the ground. He fell asleep fast in a flash.

Carberry instructed the six men who were next to him to file around his house.

He was exhausted as he and the other fell from the saddle. He mumbled, "We'll spell it in an hour," before falling into a deep sleep.

As most people feared, the hours flew by fast and men were soon back at work.

They rose to their feet. Although the brief respite was helpful, their muscles aching and the bags under their eyes warned them that it would not be enough. They had to keep going, and they knew that they would succeed.

Hartley stood still. Hartley stood back, watching the men move in front of his.

He waited for the line of pack-horses. He mused that supplies must be running low and regretted his decision to allow everyone to drink and eat as much as they wanted. His anxiety was further heightened by the slurring of empty canteens as he passed men. Their empty carry-on bags on their shoulders also raised concerns. However, he raised his lips to those passing him to express his concern and to show his confidence in his men. He felt lifted by the feeling. He called Captain Bush to inform him that he would be dancing at Tioga the next night.

Bush nodded and then bowed his tired, shaky head.

Finally, he saw the leader pack-horse. He turned around and walked back.

He was a young boy who met the lead driver and walked alongside him. He noticed that many of the horses following the boy were carrying very light loads and some had nothing on their backs. He asked the boy, "Provisions low?".
"Yes sir," the boy replied, but he was directed to give the

men all they wanted."
Hartley replied, "Oh, yes", "I know, don't worry about it." Soon, we will.

You will be able to acquire Tioga and Sheshequin, and possibly Chemung. You will find new provisions there, I promise you."

The boy suddenly said, "That's what all of us figured," and it was

The colonel's spirit was what attracted him. He added, "Rome and Carthage.". The colonel raised an eyebrow.

"The Senate decided that the best way for Rome to be protected was to carry."

The war in Africa brought the Carthaginians to the defense. "From that point onwards it was considered good defensive tactics for carrying an offensive campaign into enemy's country," said the boy.

Hartley was shocked by the reference to military tactics made by the boy. Hartley was shocked by the boy's reference to military tactics.

You wouldn't expect such insight from Philadelphians, much less from a frontier boy. He wished that some members of Congress would share his insight. He said, "Yes indeed," in reference to the boy's approval of and understanding of his tactics.

"War is never easy, especially when it comes to such high odds.

This one," the boy said, "but, but, with true faith and courage and a belief God who drives and guides us, we will emerge victorious." He nodded his head. "My Pa has always told me this."

Hartley said "Your Pa", trying to find out his identity.

He didn't know who he was referring to. He thought, "A man with great insight and high rank. He had never heard of such a man speak. He asked, "Would you name your name Butler?" with a sharp eye.

"Yes sir," the boy replied. "Lord Butler son of Colonel Zebulon Butler in Wyoming," the boy's pride was evident. "Pa likes my sister and me to read and keep up with things. He asked them to set up a route that would deliver the Courant from Connecticut. They did. After a moment of reflection, he said "Well, Pa among other things." His Pa taught him honesty.

Hartley said, "Well, he sure has done a great job with you."

said. "How old are your?" He thought back to Sweeney's story about how a Wyoming boy had assumed the commissary duties for the new battalion, which included frontiersmen, regulars, and militiamen that he commanded. However, he did not mention the name of the boy and Butler had declined to tell him about his son's participation in the expedition. Denison also had not mentioned it.

The boy replied, "Seventeen." "But I'm just equally fit and capable," he replied.

as the next!"
"Oh, no doubt, son, no doubt," Hartley said. Hartley looked back at

One of the horses that was left, contemplating whether he would prefer its back to his feet.

Lord looked up and said, "You're welcome at any of 'em," "Most officers ride, anyway, that's what Pa said." Command must be seen.

Hartley stated, "Yes, but these special circumstances are." Hartley said, "If my

Men walk, and I must also walk. It is important that men feel like they are being led in this campaign.

Lord stated, "That's a smart way to put it." "I'm sure Pa

I would agree and say the exact same."

Hartley stated, "I'm certain, also," promising to get to know.

He got to know his Wyoming counterpart better when they met face-to-face. "I'm most sure."

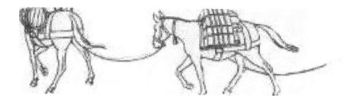

Chapter Thirty-Six

The crestfallen warriors rushed into Ester's Town, greeting them with solemn faces. They emerged from the trails and woods in small groups of threes or fours, with no more than half a dozen. After they had finished ranting about the hordes coming from the south, they mingled around looking for a pattern or reason in each others eyes. Stark looked at them all, but each was void of any thought about what the next step should be. It was all too sudden. The Yankees entered through the backdoor and no one knew how to shut it. They returned to their cabins after a while, swearing oaths in opposition to the white-eyes and praying that the Great Spirit would deliver them. Despite their promises to end the Yankee scourge, they found no relief from the greencoats who invaded the town from the North. They had heard it all before. They found that the rangers' plans did more to make their problems worse than they solved them. Each white man's boasts were met with angry grunts.

Queen Ester was seen walking amongst the angry warriors. She noticed Chief Big Man absent from their ranks, and his widow crying the most sorrowful wailings. Ester felt her grief and stopped to comfort her as warriors gathered around her, growing more furious at the sight.

Ester wept and lifted her arms to the heavens, beseeching

The heavens will intercede for them. She looked up at the sun setting behind the mountains with tear-tinted eyes. She wept openly as she looked at the green mountains. She asked, "Is she the last of her people?".
Many responded to their Queen's appeals to the Great Sky People.

The warriors shouted in protest. They stood with their spears in tight grips on their chests and swore that no white-eyes would enter the village. A few of the warriors were overcome by sheer emotion and cut their chests with sharp knives.

Ester immediately scolded the children. "Injure your white-eyes.

She said, "You are my friends!" She stood tall and regained her dignity, as she faced the last rays from the evening sun that were flooding the valley with their golden light. No! It would not be the end of her village and her husband Eghobund! His kingdom would continue as long as the water flowed and the grass grew. His widow was determined to carry his resolve from the grave. She commanded everyone to gather and then retreat to the deep glen along the Chemung River. They could defend themselves and defeat an enemy with its high walls.

Both men and women quickly gathered everything they could,

The German Flats' crestfallen prisoners were included. The horses neighed in protest as braves quickly rounded them up. There was no time to waste! They have to flee for their safety! They must flee for their lives! Even if they were not involved in the final battle, the Yankees' fury threatened everyone.

The white men's leading officer shook his head, and he mounted.

His horse yelled at his mingling soldiers to follow him to Chemung. One of his subalterns raised a protest and he turned his head to him. He asked Terry, frustrated.

Lieutenant

Terry stated. Terry said, "You should do it in his place Captain Caldwell!"

Caldwell looked down at the impudent. Caldwell retrained his horse

He was next to him, furious at being second-guessed by his men. He said, pointing towards the confused mass, "If you want to stay, do so."

Indians. "But don't expect any help from this bunch!" They're all going, and so am i!" Terry inquired.

"Captain Butler lies somewhere between here and Kanadasaga. Fine

Sir, I have your leave if you want to fetch him. At this time, I am in control and I suggest we retreat to Chemung. Maybe we might give battle in defiles between here-and-there." He turned his horse toward the north and galloped for it.

Terry looked at Caldwell's men, who were hurriedly following him.

He suddenly found himself alone amongst a sea of brown faces, terrified. He huffed and walked up the trail, looking back nervously. He knew that his capture would be from the former ranks of his service and that the neck stock around it would be loose. He felt his neck tighten and restrict him, his feet moving faster due to the sensation.

Lydia Strope ignored the white men fleeing from agitated Indians, and instead focused her attention on Lydia Strope. She looked south along the riverbank, looking for signs of her rescuers from hell. Though she thought about escaping to the south to gather her children, she reconsidered and turned her attention to her children's thoughtful eyes. She sighs and reminds herself that this is the wilderness. The trails were home to wolves, bears and rattlesnakes, as well as wolves, wolves, and panthers. They could miss the army of fast-moving soldiers, which was about a hundred miles away from her nearest civilization. The risk was greater than the chance of success. Her own life could be at risk, but her children's lives are not. Ester had been there to protect them, even though they almost starved. But at least they were able to draw the breath of life.

She turned her head in disapproval at the approaching braves.

Knowing their intentions. She quickly gathered her children, and her precious bundle of fire cake, and passed the bundle to her eldest son. She ripped down the blanket that covered the hut's entrance and wrapped her family bible in it. Anxious braves cheered "Jogo!" Jogo!"

She gathered her children and joined the ragged column.

Refugees flee the Indian village.

Under the direction of their Queen, the whole village moved north and trusted her with their lives. The Queen was familiar with the Yankees. She was aware of the rage in their hearts. She would rescue them and protect them from its horrible wrath.

Lydia trudging forward turned her head and looked behind.

She clutched the bible tightly to her chest, hoping that soldiers would come along and liberate her. Alas, they didn't come. She cried and bowed in sorrow. This could never end?

Indian women wailing and moaning in heartbreaking cries

She heard the sound of it all around her. She was free to say a silent prayer, without fear of reprisal, asking the heavens to send soldiers to rescue her and her children.

In the still night, prayers and wails drifted into nothingness.

air. The abandoned village was ringed by the howls and bellows of abandoned cattle, as well as the neighs of a few horses. The dogs were suddenly full of joy at the bounty and ate every bit of food they could find, squandering every pot and bundle.

Despite the fact that there were still a few flames in the isolated village, none of them were lit by humans.

life shone about it.

Ester's Town stood alone at night, empty of its inhabitants

Without even one shot. They were enslaved by the wrathful Yankees.

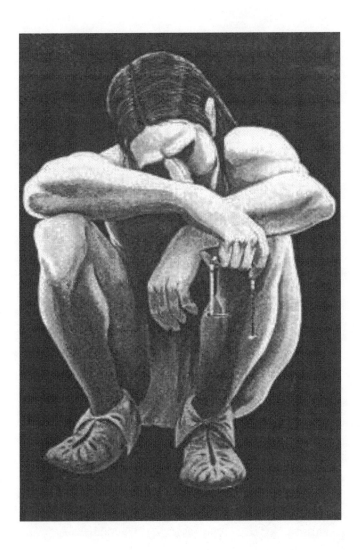

Chapter Thirty-Seven

The rifles were jolted to their shoulders by a sharp chirp, rustle of leaves, and then a sudden chirp. The scouts were able to relax as much as they were startled by the sight of the many little tails wriggling up fallen logs and underbrush, as well as their hearts. If he didn't claim an immense amount of relief, any of them would have looked foolishly at him. But, they all spoke from the terrible feeling in their stomachs.

"Chipmunks," one finally said, as he sighed under his tired eyes. "Chipmunks of all the damned things!"

Covenhoven stated, "Don't worry if they critters," now

Passing to the front of the Scouts on the steep trail, "worry for them varmints painted faces and feathers."

Slowly, the scouts resumed their march behind the brave scout in

their lead. They knew that their only chance of victory was to move fast. They quickly moved ahead in the dimming sunlight, exhausted but aware of the dangers that awaited them at every turn on the narrow trail. This was the Moravians' last section of trail that descends to Sheshequin, called the Narrow Way. They all agreed on the name.

Smaller game, such as squirrels and rabbits were also taken.

They were farther away from them as they descended the mountain trail. The Rifles moved in the right way, with an overwhelming feeling of relief every time they saw the innocent culprits making the noise.

The scouts said, "We're getting closer." "The Indians allowed these small varmints to eat the leftovers from their fields in the summer, while they hunted further away. That way when it rained, they had plenty of food for their village. They are cunning rascals.

All the advance scouts stopped for a moment to watch an

A hugely obese raccoon walks slowly along the trail, dragging it behind him. One of the raccoons whispered, "My God!" "He's fat enough for me to make a coat for my entire family!" Damn, if these Indians don't live in paradise!" One of them replied.

Covenhoven called the line back, saying "Keep it down," and pointing out

Continue down the trail to reach a flat plain beyond. Between the trees were fire flecks, silhouettes of buildings shining against their dim light. Covenhoven raised them all to his chest, forming a group around him. "I don't know how many there are or if they have all taken wing before me." He said, "All check your firelocks and get ready, call the horse at the front." He dumped some of the contents from his canteen onto the ground, much to the surprise of all those around him. He smeared the black earth on his face by swirling it in the dirt.

Many others followed his example, approving of his masking efforts.

lead. Soon, white eyes emerged from darkened faces and gave them an unnatural appearance in the pale moonlight.

Captain Carberry and his horsemen almost made it to the front as they trotted towards him.

The men collided with each other, bringing their horses to a halt just behind them. He exclaimed, "Good God, you men seem as if they popped out of the bowels the earth!" "We saw you," said barley.

Franklin and Covenhoven both made a point of putting a finger on their lips.

Motioning to Carberry to follow the trail. The fires flickered brighter.

Carberry sat down beside the scouts, dismounting. "We've

He smiled with pride and said, "It's done it!" "We have swept them under our feet unawares."

Franklin stated that the hen was the smartest creation of nature. She only cackles after the egg is laid.

Covenhoven stated, "He's right." "We have a cunning foe, who may

Do not wait for ambush to be set up near our front. "We must be careful."

Carberry nodded and mounted again. He said, "You're correct Captains." "Fine sirs, I await your orders."

Covenhoven stated, "Well, first of all we need to send an runner back to Colonel Hartley." "In the meantime we will push forwards, and I'm sure we will gain no objection from the good colonel. All are tired and feetore, and I

I am certain he wants to win the village as quickly as possible."
Franklin, Carberry and Carberry both nodded in agreement.

Covenhoven urged, "Move swiftly and quite," staring into the

The trail between them, the village, and darkens. "If we light fire from the hills, our horse will make all noise to confuse and disrupt our foe. We will attack from the front. They should run in the confusion." He took his first step forward, anxious but aware of the future. He wanted to be a role model. Their lives depended on a concerted effort from Yankee, Pennamite and regular soldiers alike. Their petty quarrels and disagreements were truly laughable in this light.

They were more energetic the closer they got to the village.

Particularly those from Wyoming, where they were scouts. They had vivid visions of the horrific battle in their minds which fueled their determination and thirst for revenge. Soon, all sense of their exhausted and aching bodies was lost. Their hands gripped the firelocks tighter. Their eyes scanned the surroundings, scanning for any movement. As they got closer to the village, the shadows around the fires became more clear. People, not just dogs, moved around the fires. Although most people sat still and watched the flames burn, one or two climbed occasionally to see the south trail.

The scouts glided through the shadows, melting into the Sheshequin Village. They encircled the fire and all those who were around it, without anyone being aware. They rose from the shadows and levelled their weapons against the shocked and scared people upon hearing Covenhoven's signal.

They were greeted with great smiles, much to their surprise. White people

People rose from their seats around the fire to run to them, overwhelmed by their presence. "Glory to God!" One of the men exclaimed, with a hint of white around his neck, "We have been delivered from savage hands by the grace of God!" "Rejoice children! Rejoice!" He ran towards the nearest Scout, and openly hugged him. Many others followed his lead.

Franklin waved one hand and said "Now, just hold on for a minute."

The grateful white people waved their men towards the cabins, while the man waving to them. "Where are the devils?"

The village's perimeter is ringing with thundering hooves

The rescuers heard a startle in their hearts. They quickly retreated to a group huddled around the fire.

Franklin called the preacher, "You!" "Answer me! "Where's the?"

devils at?"

He said, "They've all fled," trying to comfort and soothe his grieving family.

flock. "They fled at dusk with such haste that they left us by the fire. They were aware of God's promises! They knew they were near the terrible sword of God's wrath! Praise the Lord!

Franklin exclaimed, "Praise be the Lord at this, preacher." He motioned to his men to continue their inspection of each cabin, always mindful of their wily foe.

One of the Scouts hurried forward and examined all the faces quickly.

The huddled masses. When none of the faces he recognized, he reacted in dismay. He asked the preacher, "Are they still around Ester's Town or Tioga Point?".

"I don't know what lies upriver my dear man. Only that God knows."

"Bring this flock of worthy souls out of the hands of the savages," he said, bowing in prayer.

He said, "More worthy souls lay upriver preacher," "I know."

That fer sure!" He ran from the fire and began to search all the cabins. He stumbled towards the fire in despair and collapsed from exhaustion. He gasped for Lydia, his dear family.

Franklin stated, "It'll all be alright Boss." "We'll head there at first."

light."

Before Boss could speak, Covenhoven declared "First light hell." He knelt next to the man in crestfallen, and pats his shoulder.

Carberry galloped to the fire and reined his horse back on its hind legs

haunches. He asked, "Who are these poor souls?".

"Just the faithful servants the Lord delivered from Satan"

"Wrath," replied the preacher to the horseman.

Carberry quickly counted the heads. He said, "Fifteen," and looked around.

The river was dark. He asked, "How many poorer people await deliverance up river?".

"Perhaps more," a commanding voice broke into the

air. Colonel Hartley emerged from shadows strong and stout. He smiled and looked with comforting eyes at the freed souls who were huddled around the fire. Troops rushed behind him to search the cabins.

The preacher exclaimed, "Oh, Praise dear God, an officer with high rank." "Sent to deliver our souls from evil!"

Hartley looked up at the north trail and said "Well,"

I am aware of that, but you are delivered. I trust you will be right about God's hand being with our needs, as I fear that we may need all the help possible.

Boss Strope rose above his grief and plodded up the trail to north. Hartley was the object of anxious eyes.

He told the Scouts and Carberry to "Go on", if they felt up to it. Ester's Village will be next after we've captured Sheshequin. Grab all that you can and throw away everything you don't have! We will see to it. Plunder can be recovered and livestock needs to be reared. If you need assistance, please let us know. Do not go any further than Ester's Town. I fear Chemung is too far away this night. We will see what happens on the morrow."

Most of the Light Horse and Scouts walked up the hill.

They quickly disappeared into the darkness of the forest, following the trail. They were no longer tired and walked lively on the trail until the early hours of the morning, fueled by their hunger for the hunt.

"Gentlemen! I will have a strong security guard posted this evening, the

Parole shall be a 'victory'," Hartley said to the last scouts climbing up the trail. "The countersign shall not be 'or death!

Weep to Ester if she is found this evening, for there was no mercy.

Their hearts were filled with a desperate thirst for justice. It was the only way to quench their desperate thirst for justice.

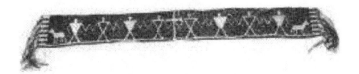

Chapter Thirty-Eight

The Light Horse galloped forward in the darkness and swooped down on Ester's Town. They outnumbered the scouts and galloped through Ester's Town, scattering the dogs. They raced to the cabin doors, kicked them in one foot from their mounts, and carried pistols, carbines and swords at all that moved.

Fire flecks are still smoldering flames and embers in the fire

The shadows cast by the pits that dot the village's walls are eerie. One of the horsemen reached for a pine knot that was lying by one of the cabins, and bent down to make a fire in the pit. The man's determined and grimy face was illuminated by the pine knot, which glowed to life. He kicked his horse's back, and he galloped toward the nearest cabin.

Carberry called him "No!" "There is still plunder in them.

The foot soldiers will take care of it! All shall be set ablaze after they have cleared it!" He galloped toward the north end, the Light Horse following. Their trot was accelerated by a series of shots throughout the night.

Two horsemen sat on their horses, trying to reinvigorate.

They held their positions while trying to load the guns into their hands. One of them said that about a half-dozen of them had scurried up and down the trail. Captain, I got a few shots but it was not enough!

Carberry rode up the trail with a rod, and stared up at it.

Own pistol. He looked back at the village, anxiously. He turned to the north trail, noting that the scouts were coming in from the south. He said, "The foot's here!" It's a great night for a hunt with foxes! Let's go!" They then roared up the path. Soon, the thundering sound of their hooves vanished into the dark foreboding.

Boss Strope raced through the Indian village, slamming

He opens the doors with his rifle butt, and immediately twirls it around, ready to kill any wild animal lurking in the shadows. He saw no faces. He had visions of Lydia's smile in his head. He must find her! He must find them! He continued to walk, eventually falling on the ground in exhaustion. He rolled over and cursed his exhausted body, asking for strength. He saw the silhouette of a tree-lined riverbank in his eyes. He sensed Lydia instinctively. He rose to his feet and dragged his long rifle behind.

He fell into the hut headfirst, looking madly for the shadows.

Any sign of his children or wife. He was astonished to discover a familiar but faint odor. He smelled the faint scent! It was his swear word! He crawled from the cabin and fell down the bank half expecting to find his wife and children at the bottom. He was greeted only by a handful of canoes. He kicked them with his feet and sent one into the current. He finally gave up, and fell to the sandy beach.

"Wait!" A voice called from the bank high above. "We might need..."

them canoes!"
Covenhoven plunged down a bank, splashing in water.

The canoe was barely caught just as it reached the main current. He pulled the canoe back and threw it onto the shore. He collapsed, gasping and grunting.

Boss murmured, "They've taken it," to him. They were just

Here, I can feel them! "I can smell 'em!" He attempted to get up, but he collapsed again. "Damn Copperheads stole 'em from under my nose!"

"No, damn it!" Covenhoven said. "You've done everything you can!" No

one could've done better!"

Boss sobbed, "I shouldn't have left 'em, damnit." "But Denison

They promised to return them! I had to travel for him and his troops. I had to warn

Wyoming!"

Covenhoven stated, "It's not his fault, nor yours!"

He walked along the beach, his tired body fighting against every movement. He and his rangers could do more than him. It was a difficult trek of thirty miles through the wilderness. He was amazed at the feat. There was nothing better. He looked at his fellow who was in a state of shock. He said, "Get hold of yourself. He groaned, "We shall find them on Monday.".

"No," Boss said. "That half-breed Ester is taking them to Fort Niagara, or worse!" I'm going back up to the Hudson to gather my people. They'll find them!" His head dropped to the sand. He closed his eyes immediately and fell into deep sleep despite his pain.

Covenhoven sat down and listened. From the other side, a slight rustle was heard.

The night was still quiet in the village and there were no more shots. He took a deep breath and fought to keep his eyes open. He knew that if he did, he would also fall asleep. He mumbled, "Not yet," to his aching body. "Not yet!"

He sat up and looked at the swirling waters below him. A fish

He jumped and made a splash right in front of them, giving him a start. The slight energy boost from the start gave him the opportunity to grab one of Boss' feet in the water. He pulled it from the water and slowly rose. He took a sip from the nearly empty canteen and walked back to the village.

He was greeted by exhausted men with bloodshot eyes. He struggled.

He walked towards the fire pits, which were blazing with heat from the plentiful supply of wood. He bent down and picked up a burning pine knot as he walked towards the cabin at the village's center. The door to the fine hewn log structure was surrounded by an ornamental porch. He reasoned that this was the home of someone of great importance. It was a Queen! He opened the door and prepared to throw the firebrand in it. His movements were immediately stopped by a hand on his arm.

Franklin asked Franklin, "Don't think we should wait until we have had a look around?".
Covenhoven replied, "It's the fiend Ester's place for certain." "It

must burn!"
Franklin's eyes widened at the sight of this name. "All the more

He explained why it was important not to pass it on until we have had the chance to examine it.".

Covenhoven said, "Be my guest sir," taking a step.

backward. His stomach felt churned. His legs cramped. He was unable to sleep.

Another Wyoming man said, "None would want it to burn as we."

He said this as he walked up to the men at the doorway. "As well the one who occupies it," he stated. He kicked through the skins and blankets that lay on the floor, rifling through the contents of each hearth. He stumbled across something in the middle of the floor, fumbling in the dim lighting. The idol was a grotesque representation of something from neither hell nor heaven and it fell from its place on the stump at the center of the cabin. Repelled by the sight, he looked at it through tired eyes and ran back through the door.

Franklin asked Franklin, "Well Roswell?".

"There is nothing in there except something from neither this nor that side."

Roswell Franklin stated, "Heaven or hell," "Burn it, let your stench foul the nostrils Satan!"

Covenhoven tossed a firebrand in the door and fell back.

It. Roswell Franklin followed him and threw his pine knot into the door. Soon, smoke began to roll through the doors. The fire lit up the room, shining through thick columns and billowing black smoke. The gathering of scouts, rangers elicited muffled cheers.

Franklin stated, "That's it for tonight." "We'll wait until morning."

at first light. There are cattle out there, and we have our own plunder around this place. After we have reclaimed everything, we will burn it.

The exhausted men did not raise a protest. Some were already there

Collapsed and snored in fire pits, on the sides of cabins and inside them.

Covenhoven, who was barely able keep his eyes open, said that "We'll have to watch."

Keep your eyes open. "Parole means 'victory'. Countersign is or death.

Franklin observed, "Me here and Roswell will see to it," Franklin stated.

The flames lighten the mountains and reflect off of the Susquehanna. "Waited a long time for it, would love to see it burn."

Roswell stated, "It's true, I wish they all" Roswell, raising his hand.

His chest with the rifle. "And I would very much love to fall one of those who murdered

Captain Stewart, should any of them be foolish enough to show their face!"

Covenhoven murmured, "Prisoners," before collapsing beside a

fire pit. "Prisoners. We must know the strength of the rats and their plans. Prisoners." He shook his head for a moment before suddenly coming back to life. "Wake me, and I'll spell it in a bit. Pay attention to the horse. They'll return. Keep your prisoners in check!" He fell asleep again, his snoring adding to the noise pollution.

Roswell, as he walked towards the embassy, said "We'll be seeing about prisoners."

The village's north end. "We'll see exactly what they saw about Wyoming prisoners!"

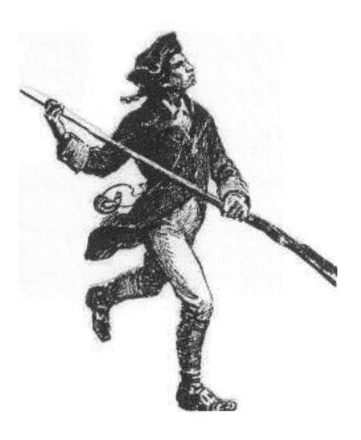

Chapter Thirty-Nine

Ester looked down at the jewels on her horse. Each of the gems, taken from her victims and reminiscing about her individual circumstances, reminded Ester. On her people's lonely trek through the wilderness, each of these memories haunted her. All seemed to be for nothing at the moment.

The souls who followed her to the glen were now ruled by silence. There were no more crying children, no more weeping widows, and no more whooping warriors.

She had originally thought she would lead them to Chemung but changed her mind.

It was afraid it would be the Yankee's true target. There was too much bloodshed between them now to fight for anything other than the end. The war seemed to be one of annihilation. It was a terrible, complete war.

Her eyes widened to see the raven feathers that were all around her.

horse's mane. The horse's mane swayed and moved naturally because a woman had spent great effort to dress her Queen's horse. Their bluish-black color sparkled in the dim light of the moon. They were so beautiful that she lost herself in them and fell into a trance. Beauty was needed to soothe her thoughts, as she had no other thoughts but to think of the horrible.

Her horse stumbled upon a stone, and she neighed breaking the silence

The mood. Their Queen was surrounded by a sea of eyes. She shook her head and waved at them to continue, then reined her horse along the trail.

She felt something brush along her leg, and she looked down at the hair.

Whirling in the wind. She reached out to grab a string of fourteen scalps as retribution for her son's death by the Yankees. One fell to the ground. She didn't dismount to retrieve the item. In vengeance, too much blood had flowed from the palm of her hand. It did not help her grief. It seemed to only increase the pain. Oh, Gencho, my son! He was her last hope for Chief Eghobound. She let her tears flow, turning her back to the Indians ahead of her. They were already in enough pain. She didn't want to increase their anxiety.

The trees echoed with the sound. A few raised their heads.

Others let out an anxious gasp and walked steadfastly ahead, disregarding the strange noise. A few warriors raced back towards the noise, looking into the trail's darkness behind them. The warriors looked around, then saw their queen sitting still on her mare of great black. They thought that Ester had taken the horse from Wyoming and made a loss of some Wyoming horse flesh. One of them saw the hair and bent down. Ester was still looking at him as he gingerly lifted the hair and gave it to him.

Ester quickly wiped her eyes, and she accepted the scalp.

It was tied to the string by others. She sucked hard at her grief and cracked a half smile to the brave.

The brave didn't speak but he only looked deeply into her eyes. His

The white flag of a deer trail crossing behind them caught his attention. The relief gave way to anguish, and he sighed again. He looked at the Queen with hollow eyes and sighed.

Ester said, "Jogo Roland," to the staring face with the pot-marked mark.

She looked up at her with a deep, soulful gaze. His eyes begged for an explanation, but she didn't have one. She turned her eyes away from him, and began to trot up the trail.

Roland Montour stopped, turned to the braves, and stared

Continue down the trail. They noticed a dim light just above the trail's crest that caught their attention. They understood what it meant. They lost everything they had.

Roland fell to his knees and began to pound the ground. Throwing

He lowered his head and let out a long, mournful cry. John, his brother, walked slowly toward him and knelt beside him. Tears of anger and anguish were fluttering down their cheeks as John bows his head.

Ester slowed her horse and then turned around to face them. She called out to her brothers in their native language, "John, Roland! My blood!" "Rise! Be strong! This one is gone, but our day will come again. We will see Seneca when he comes! They will help us drive Yank-ee from this land for ever! Par le fer et par le feu! Avoir de l'estomac!"

The bravest of them turned and walked solemnly towards the ruins.

Retracting line of souls. John helped Roland to rise, and they both walked slowly past the Queen. Roland noticed that the Queen didn't follow his lead and he ordered a pair braves to return to her.

Ester ignored their warnings and pushed her horse up the steep side.

trail. The dark forest was her constant companion, and she finally reached the summit of the mountain. She was accompanied by brave men who kept up the pace.

She retrained her horse to a small clearing in the trees and gazed down

To the valley below. On either side, the braves gazed down at the valley below, sharing the same grief as their queen. They all watched the embers of a single fire flicker below them. They were relieved to see only one building burn, but they knew it was Queen Ester's castle.

Ester sat silently watching the flames, and then suddenly remembered all she had.

forgotten in her haste. Her husband had made a prayer idol with his own hands. It was meant to symbolize all he knew about the Great Spirit. It was kept in a prominent place at the castle's center in her village. It was fitting because he was the center of her universe, even after she died. Her universe was now nothing.

All those who had walked this path for so many years were left with nothing.

They were there hundreds of years ago. It all went up in flames, she realized. Everything she had preserved from that past was now ashes. All were set on fire by a new intruder, one unlike any Indian nation. The white-eyes. After watching the Moravian missionaries read from the book, she thought back to the bark tablets Neolin had made. He had spoken his word around the Tioga great fire to many great chiefs, but none greater than the great Ottawa Chief Pontiac. Neolin, who stood for many years at the southern entrance of the

Iroquois Confederacy and resented all the treacherous white eyes. He was the one who had brought dust into New Castle's eyes, Penn's negotiator. New Castle believed in the great power of medicine men and ran back to

Philadelphia, to expire one month later while Neolin's power was being mumbled about. The wampum about this story now rose to the heavens as flames. She hoped that the smoke they inhaled into the great skies would carry the magic back to Neolin, and all the other great men who had made Tioga their home. Maybe then they would be able to help the world beyond. All they had ever been was now gone in the face the unrelenting tides of the white-eyes. It was a horrible thought that she couldn't bear to think about.

The braves looked up at the Queen of Heaven, and noticed glittering tears.

Her cheeks were reflected in the moonlight. Both of them turned and gazed at the flickering flames and silhouettes of the avenging demonics in their light. They both swear an oath to revenge in their native languages.

The Queen looked at them and suddenly felt nauseated.

The sickening cry for revenge rolling from their lips. She snatched the scalps, and then she jerked her fingers back as if they were smoldering from hatred. The Wyoming Yankee was only motivated by her revenge when she took the scalps. She saw the futility of the whole thing and believed it was a vicious cycle that would never end, until the universe ended.

She shook her head and muttered Eghobund's name.

In recognition of the great chief, the braves' eyes lit up in admiration.

The rage that burns in their hearts.

She yelled "Jogo" to the angry braves as she reined her horse back

To the trail. She didn't turn around to see the pain behind her. She stared straight ahead, her eyes fixed on the pain of her family. It demanded her complete attention. She allowed the darkness to engulf her troubled memories, and she hoped they would remain forever in the darkness beyond.

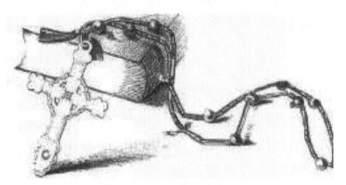

Chapter Forty

Roswell Franklin wandered through the cabins at the village's northern edge. Roswell Franklin walked through the cabins at the northern edge of the village, where the intense fire from Queen Elizabeth's castle sank into the shadows of trees. He sat down, looking at the trees for any sign of movement, and held his rifle in his hands. He looked around for Captain Franklin, who was supposedly on guard duty with him. But he gave up after an hour.

The air was filled with snorts, grunts, and occasionally, lip smacks.

him. He ignored the other men for making such a racket, while he concentrated on his duty. He could not help but think of the exhausted souls of his fellow soldiers. But he knew someone had to be there.

He took a huge gulp to keep his head still and try to avoid bobbing.

From his canteen. He was shook by the force of the harsh rye whiskey. He suddenly remembered that they were looking for prisoners. He carefully scanned the entire village and paced around it, looking into the trees lit by the great fire. He thought about how he would get the village and grab a Rebel's hair. He focused his attention on a low ridge to the west. It was dotted with scrub oaks. A few cattle grazed the plain beyond it. One could follow the ridge to the village's edge, then spurt out and club a sentry. He would be stunned at what he had done. It was a remarkable feat that could be achieved by a warrior.

Slowly, he walked to the edge. He found a nice clump of

He melted into the brush, watching closely the other side of the ridge, and scanning the perimeter. He reasoned that if they were coming, then this was the way. This is the trap. You will soon have some fun if you remain still.

He took off his wide-brimmed slouch cap and sat it down.

He was right next to him. He felt the mud on his skin. The mud felt dry but still held onto his cheeks. He sat down and placed his hands on the rifle in front of him. He tried to reduce the size of his whites as much as possible by focusing on his eyes. Amazing eyes were the mark of the Indians, who were wily hunters in the forest. He told himself he would, because his life depended on it.

He fought against his heavy eyelids and moved his knee to the side.

He could see a sharp, protruding stone on the ground in front. He placed his right knee on top of it and applied just enough pressure to keep his eyes open. Sometimes, pain can be a good partner in hunting, especially with this foe.

He sat and listened to the crackle of fire and occasional beam.

Falling from the cabin and watching as a flash of light appeared in the air, when the beam fell. A tree high up on the mountain rang out with the sound of an owl. He listened attentively and relaxed when the owl took the wing. The owl then swooped down onto him. He saw its enormous wings beat in the wind as it rose into the night sky. The long snake moved slowly and rolled its head against its talons. He watched the snake disappear into the trees, then he lowered his gaze and looked around. He began to slowly draw his tomahawk from his belt. He placed the tomahawk in a convenient place while holding his rifle in one hand.

He noticed a slight movement in the upper right corner of his eyes.

ridge. He sat still, watching the specter. The tall Indian grass that topped the ridge moved slightly but not from the ground. He looked in the direction the movement was taking him, but failed to see anything in the darkness. He saw more grass move, but only a little. He took a deep, slow breath. His white hands clutched his rifle. The faint glow of light from the fire at his rear dancing among the tall grass was all he could see. He was only a few yards from the grass that had moved for what seemed like a lifetime. He was afraid someone would be watching him closely.

The owl, his old friend, flew down from the tree and flapped it.

He had huge wings that extended above the grass and brush along the ridge. It was ignored by him. He did not ignore his foe. His foe did not. The whites of his pair of eyes turned toward the sky for a heartbeat. After careful examination, the rest was found in the grass and brush below.

He cursed his breath and did not want to betray anyone.

His presence was a sign of his close enemy. He pressed his knee against the rock. He must sharpen all his senses! He must be alert He should not slack off!

His whites stared at him with their pair of eyes.

He remained stationary for the longest time before turning his back, much to his relief. He was still rigid and wished for courage to move, but he only walked a few more feet before he moved. He should know if others followed. He should only strike when certain of winning.

The brave moved their hands along the ground, then they moved their other hand.

His body was covered in black paint, making him look like a shadow. He crawled slowly and painfully. He had to reach the top of the ridge before he could strike. At least one white eye would see his anger. He felt better the more he passed that spot, which made the nape of the neck tingle. He sensed something there even though his eyes were blank. When suddenly stars appeared in his vision, he moved one hand forward. He fell, feeling his hands loosening all their strength. He lost his knife and tomahawk.

He was furious and flung his hands at the unseen demon.

He shook his head and his fingers caught some flesh. He dug into them with all of his might. Another thud followed. A scream was the next. Another blow to his head caused his neck to bend unnaturally. His throat was flooded with a metallic taste. All went dark.

Roswell shouted, "Damn!" and threw down his clubbed rifle. Roswell instinctively grabbed his bleeding arm and stared at the brave, motionless before him. He looked down and kicked the Indian's arm, looking for the knife that had tore his flesh. He crouching down, picked up the knife and tomahawk of the brave, noting that no blood was visible on them. He was frustrated and ready to tie the hands of the brave. Under the fingers of the brave, something curled up and dangled. Skin! He said, "Damn it all," wrapping his bleeding arm in a rag. "I hate to imagine what he would do with that tomahawk. The accursed rascal."

He moved to his rear and he flung his head to the face of a new scene.

threat. Boss Strope stood with his rifle at his shoulder and aimed at the brave. His bloodshot eyes were glaring at him. He moved a few steps forward.

Roswell, picking up his rifle, said "Damn it!" Roswell said, picking up his rifle.

"Avoid attracting attention to a man like this, especially in these parts"

Boss looked at him and noticed the blood running down his legs.

arm. He asked, "Did you get rascal?".
Roswell stated, "Ain't nothing." "Well, we got a prisoner, but if'n he lives, that is."
Boss stated, "The next time he'll breath is in the fiery pits and hell." He aimed his rifle at the Indian's head and pulled the trigger. In the still air, a hollow click rang. Boss exclaimed, raising his weapon and pulling the hammer back. It failed again.

Roswell replied, "Now, just hold onto." "That buck is my prisoner."

Boss stated, "If you have a hankering after his hair, it's yours!".
He threw aside his useless rifle and drew his long knives. He sat down on his back and grabbed the short strip of hair that ran along the middle of his head.

He quickly let the hair slip through his fingers. He said, "Damn Indian's hair is full of grease!" and wiped his pants before picking up the hair. He moaned loudly.

Roswell stated, "He's still breathing." "Colonel needs a prisoner. Boss, you should back off.

Roswell Franklin, you take care of your place Roswell Franklin. I will take care of mine. This buck is most likely Lydia's blood! They are mine! All of them! Boss yelled, "Damn these Copperheads!" He placed the blade on the neck of the Indian who was groaning. "You fine-haired rascal! "Get ready to meet your maker!"

"Strope!" A voice called from behind the men. "Roswell's

right! We need a prisoner! "You should drop that blade!" The click sound in the air.

Boss asked, "Would you kill a white man to save a damn savage?" Boss asked.

He didn't pay attention to the voice. His bloodshot, bulging eyes were fixed on the brave. His shaking hand stopped him from pulling the blade across his neck by quickly reaching for his shoulder. He was aided by another hand, who gently took the knife from him. In amazement, he looked up at the man in front of him.

John Franklin smiled at them. He said, "It'll all be fine, Boss." It's been a difficult time for us all but we still have to follow orders. You know that we aren't out yet. This Indian could have a lot to tell us about our current situation. You might even be able to tell us about your people."

Boss heard the last words echo through his mind. "You're right," he

He backed away from the brave, he said. He dropped the knife and raised both hands to his face, staring blankly at his hands. "This war makes us all murders."

Franklin stated, "Ain't no murder in the line-of-duty." Pulling a length

He took rawhide out of his pocket and bent down to tie the hands of the brave.

Covenhoven, speaking with others, said "Good job."

The commotion woke him up. He patted John Franklin on his shoulder, while looking at Strope with his own eyes. He asked, "Do you think that he'll be alright?".

Franklin stated, "Hard to know." "Hard to know if any of us will escape."

This is the same way we entered it. It is the heart of the demon.

Roswell was looking over at Covenhoven. He stood straight, but

He looked exhausted that a breeze of wind could easily knock his over. Roswell, here's my spelling. Get some sleep. It's going to be very important. You did a great job. The colonel will be proud."

"Pride, hell! He can have it!" Roswell said that Boss should have had his way and stumbled back towards the village. He stumbled to a nearby cabin. He found a bear skin inside it and collapsed from exhaustion. He exclaimed, "Damn skin smells terrible!" It was just like a Copperhead. He said,

"Everything smells like hell!" and tossed it aside. He sat down and fell asleep instantly.

Covenhoven screamed, "This is hell", as he looked at the faint glow.

The sun is beginning to rise over the mountains to its east. "And when the sun comes up, we will gather all the plunder that we can, and all the rest will be burned to the fire like hell!"

Chapter Forty-One

Captain Carberry watched as the sun's dimming glow teased the eastern treetops. He moved back and forth before his exhausted horse, looking at the small Indian village where his horsemen lived. The cool morning breeze pushed everything still standing, except for the trees that swayed in the branches. He reasoned that the scouts should have stayed at Ester's Town. He didn't blame them, and he was proud of the strong but sore saddle men of his Light Horse. He had a back problem just like theirs but he didn't complain.

He could only picture the pain of footsore scouts trying to get each step. They all performed admirably. He looked at the pouch and walked over to his fellow soldiers. Some sat groggily on the ground, others walked up to their horses. Some remained still silent on the ground with their horses' reins tied to their hands, so they could mount quickly in an emergency. A few horses raised their arms and jerked their heads to wake up their exhausted masters.

Carberry took out a map and laid it on the ground. He tapped a spot on the map with his finger and said, "We are here," to those around him. He turned to the north and said, "Shawnee Village." "Chemung Village can be found just a few kilometers away!"

One of the men stated, "I don't believe any of these foot followed, sir.".

Carberry stated, "Yes, it would appear, but saddle sore certainly is different from footsore." He took a quick sip from his canteen. The canteen was almost empty. He eagerly ate a slice of ash cake out of his bag. The pieces fell all over the place. He said, "That's how the Indians work." They are scattered all over and can strike from any place at any time. They can be defeated only by a determined pursuit, cold camps, or sure-shots.

A man said, "Well, so far so well.".

Carberry said, "It will be full light soon," as he rose and folded the fabric.

map. "I hope you all have had some rest, and that the guard was spelled. We ride again today, probably harder than we have so far."

His response: "The men can handle it, sir. But the horses are almost played out."

sergeant reported. "Fodder in this area is very scarce." He moved towards one of the wild grapevines that was clinging to a nearby tree. It was nibbled by a horse. "They would not have anything if it wasn't for wild grapes or the scrub under the trees. The Shesequin Indian grass is too rough to be used for anything other than a broom. All the rest is wild rye that's not good for horses. We must find good English grass pastures.

Carberry stated, "Yes, Sergeant, I am aware," "I

I believe the Ester's flats had some promise. We saw the livestock moving about as we swept through her Town.

"We need to let them eat.

Sergeant, that is the problem.

Carberry nodded toward the trail. "We need to take a look at the trail right now.

He took a long glance at Chemung and then he climbed onto the saddle of his horse. "I will take two men with us, keep a strong watch posted here, and let the horses eat as much as they can until I return, which should happen soon."

The sergeant shook his head and said "Yes sir," before putting on his hat. "What if there were scouts?"

show up?"

"I don't think they will. They're all exhausted. I

Dare I say that the good colonel, all of them, are still at Sheshequin right now. They have been outpaced by our mounts' four feet. It has been a combination of our enthusiasm for fighting that has taken us to their front. We should not withdraw without seeing our enemies about Chemung, by the grace of God.

"No sir. We should not."

"Nor shall we."

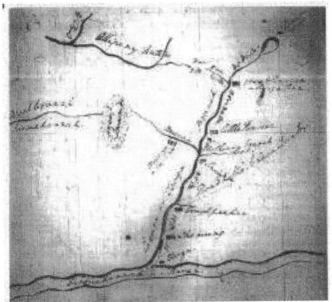

A map of Tioga Point drawn by General Washington in 1778.

Chapter Forty-Two

Captain Carberry was stunned by the sight in front of him. He glanced back at the two horsesmen who were accompanying him, and waved for them to slow down. He got up and walked away, handing his horse's reins over to the nearest horseman. He gingerly crawled forward and sat down behind a small bush at the top of a mountain, looking below.

> One of the horsemen carefully mounted and passed the reins to the other.

He walked over to his horse and ignored his protest. He walked silently towards his leader, leaving his disgruntled companion to tend to the horses. His eyes grew larger than those of the captain. In the early morning light, dozens of cabins dotted the plain below. Many fires produced smoke that hung in the air. The corral north of the village was overflowing with horses. The Chemung River, to the left of the village, sparkled in the early morning sun. The riverbanks were graced by ancient trees and great overshadowing. Behind the trees, there were many green, lush, and round fields of squash, beans, and corn. Fine English grasses grew from the river to the village's edge. The village was alive and vibrant, with many people running around the corrals and fire pits. The brightly colored clothing of Indian women was mixed with green coats and hunting shirts.

The soldier stated, "They seem excited.".
Carberry: "Yes, I'm afraid it is because our little force,"

He counted the hunting shirts and green coats. He was followed by the soldier.

"Must have at least two hundred seventy Tories down

there," the soldier said.
Carberry nervously looked at Carberry and said "Closer than three hundred."

He can be seen all around the mountain, as well as behind him. "We need to be careful, there is no telling what might pop out of the forest, so close to their nests. Keep the horses quiet.

The soldier raised a spyglass to ask, "What's it?"

He squinted his eyes. He pointed out a group of horses that were trotting towards the village along the north trail. Indian children and their dogs fled to safety. The haughty group was followed by many angry women who hurled scorns and fists. They retrained their horses before a tall, green-colored man and plopped down from their saddles just in time to stop their horses.

The horse soldier replied, "In a hurry. whoever they are.".
Carberry said "Here," and he gave him the glass. He sat down below.

He sat down on a nearby bush and placed the spyglass on top of a large, flat stone. Then he focused on the rangers. He observed the new arrivals of horsemen, particularly the small, wiry ones, and he waved contemptuously at them. The exaggerated movements and manner of the wiry man betrayed his self-importance and pride. Carberry watched him for a while longer before slowly lowering his glass. He said, "Walter Butler it's," "Indian Butler is our son and true traitor to the cause if there ever was one."

"Are your sure sir?" the soldier inquired, rubbing his hands together.

Eyes to protect them from the sun.
"Look at how he moves and banters around like a Banny rooster. It is hard to believe that such a small frame could hold such a large head. He is cocky, arrogant and full of himself. It is only a good thing he is down there, and not his father. Otherwise they would likely already be marching for us."

"Do you think that he knows our true number?"

"No, or he'd march. Even the most vile coward would march.

marche if they could see the real state of affairs."

"Lucky for us he does not, sir."
"Luck is something that one creates for himself."

Captain Carberry stood and stepped carefully to the other side.

bush. For a few seconds he stared at each section, trying to remember the layout of the land and what it was. He said that he had a few hundred men more and a couple of small cannons to make this village and the surrounding areas a total destruction. Ah, to once be properly armed and provisioned!

They were alerted by a commotion in central village

again. He was a huge chief with a barrel-chest and so tall that he towered above Indians and whites. He was joined by a growing number of warriors who gathered around him to join in the war whoops.

The soldier replied, "That is trouble." "He seems like one who means."

business and may not be afraid of the number of challenges he will face. Seneca must be his name. They will be incited by him, without doubt. We are on his land, and we know the land and how it can be fought."

Carberry felt dreadful. Carberry slowly turned his attention to

The sun was already high above the trees, and the sky. He said, "We've outstayed our welcome." "We should report as soon as possible to the colonel."

Both men moved away from the bush after the soldier nodded.

Watching the ground below to see if there was any sign they were being spotted. They quickly jumped into the saddle and backed up to the man who was riding the horses. The soldier who was watching the horses quickly mounted his own horse. He didn't ask for explanations, as the fear in the eyes of each man betrayed everything he wanted to know. Before turning his mount, he adjusted his pistols, saber and carbine so they were ready for action at a moment's notice.

They walked their horses slowly down the hill at first.

Mountain, be careful not to disturb any bush or twig. Their wide-eyed eyes absorbed every movement. They listened to every sound. All their fears were broken by the sight of the trail ahead. They rushed down the trail, breaking it under their mad hooves as they tried to get away.

They would die if they were caught. This certainty pushed the spur into horses' flanks, and the whip fell mercilessly on their backs. They could only go full speed until the dreadful ache in their hearts faded away.

They had seen the enemy and were able to see his great numbers and fade away.

They will see their life come back to life before their eyes. They felt empty with this knowledge. However, it was only a temporary feeling that would fade as they moved further away.

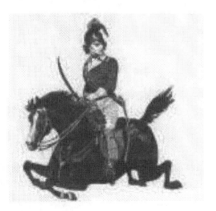

Chapter Forty-Three

Colonel Hartley dropped the biscuit in his hand and looked towards the sound of the north's thudding hooves. He abruptly got up from the fire he had shared with Captain Bush, and put his hat on. He walked towards the village guards after checking his pistols. Bush was next.

Some soldiers came to life as they groggily walked about them.

The sight of the plunder being brought in by others from their cabins. This invigorated many others from their tired sleep around the village.

Every eye, whether it was focused on plundering or not, looked towards the horizon.

The huddled prisoners were the most anxious. They held on to each other, looking at the preacher for comfort, his only offering being a quick prayer from his anxious lips.

Hartley told them all to "Be Still". All is well. It's probably just

Our Light Horse. "Eh Captain Bush?"

"Most likely, sir," Bush answered, nonetheless quickening his

Just like the colonel, march to the sound and rhythm of the hooves. He walked a few paces and whispered to the colonel, "Should we not assemble our troops?"

Hartley replied, "No, my man, my man." Hartley said, "They are already half-out of."

Their skulls were filled with worry, particularly for the poor souls that we freed last night. Don't worry, if you see any mischief, I am sure that we will all tackle it with ...". He stopped and inspected the plume of feathers on Carberry's leather cap. "See? It is Carberry with two men."

Bush declared, "My God," "Where are the other?"

"We will find out by their hard riding.

"We are." The colonel stopped right behind the sentries, who stood poised with their weapons at the ready. He waited for the horsemen, folding his arms.

The sentries moved forward a little bit, calling out "Victory!"

the horsemen.
Carberry and his men rode steadily towards the colonel.

He ignored the sentries. He yanked his hat off and slapped his horse's flanks with the hat, ignoring all the sentries.

The sentries stood firm and raised their rifles above their bodies.

Blocking the advance of the horsemen. One of them called "Victory!" again.

Carberry ignored them and slapped his horse with his hat again.

They quickly moved to block the horses. They were able to get away from the horses.

To block their rifles, they hold their guns lengthwise.

Carberry halted his horse at the last second.

You couldn't help but to plunge into the guards. The sentries were unable to resist the temptation of dirt flying from their hooves.

They didn't move a muscle.

Carberry shouted "What?" "Are you crazy!?" !"

"Victory!"
Carberry looked confused and mumbled, "or death," before he was spurred.

his horse forward.

The sentries pushed the horses back, forcing them to retreat.

Carberry shouted, "Look here, square-headed Yankee!" "Make

way!"

The sentry, wearing a red cloth tied to his shoulders, stared indefiantly

at the captain. He said, "Victory!" again.

Carberry grated his teeth and mumbled "or death" again.

One of the sentries asked, "What was that Private Terry?".
"Sounded like a bad wind blowing from some Pennamite's

The private replied, "Backside!" "We best get down wind."

Carberry exclaimed, "You stubborn Yankee rascals!" "Make way for once!"

The sentries didn't move.

"Colonel!" Carberry finally shouted, past all the sentries, "I Have!"

pertinent information! This is a foolish game!

Hartley didn't say a word and silently considered the anger among.

these men. They were kept apart by a truce that Congress had ordered after the last battle at Rampart Rocks in December Seventeen Sixty-Five. These very men faced off on the opposite side in that battle-of-men. Two hundred fifty Yankees defeated a seven hundred fifty Pennamite invasion force. Some Yankees were only equipped with pitch forks, scythe knives and poles. Due to depredations by both sides, the bitter Yankee-Pennamite War still pulsed through their veins. Their mutual enemy was all that united them. A cause, a cause forcing their differences aside, is what ties them together. He chose to keep their faith in the common cause that unites even bitter foes.

He said, "They are only concerned with their duty, Captain." "Give

Give Sergeant Baldwin the countersign, and everything will be fine. And be very quick about it! Both of you should know that the enemy is out there and not here! Keep America in your thoughts! "My good men, she is greater than all our petty differences!"

Carberry shouted "Or death!" Bending his entire torso forward, Carberry screamed.

and spattering on the sentries with his spittle.

Baldwin smartly took his place, saying, "Very good sir.".

Carberry murmured, "Damn square-headed Yankee vagabonds."

Under his breath. He was disgusted and whipped his horse through the sand.

Baldwin asked, "Did Terry hear anything?".

Jonathan Terry stated, "Just that foul Pennamite winds again." "Perhaps he should smoke some, relieves what's cooped-up even the tightest buttocks."

Hartley tried to keep a smile from appearing on his face by shaking his head.

towards the sentries.

They took the hint and returned to their duties.

Carberry screamed, "Damn these fools," and he plopped down from the

Place your saddle in front the colonel. "There's a time and place for formalities, and it's not here. They thought I was Indian Butler! Indian Butler

"Now, Captain, they're trying their best to keep proper

Hartley stated that despite our military bearing, we remain an army no matter where it is located.".

Captain Spalding, Colonel Denison suddenly appeared

Carberry was forced to control his anger at the two powerful Yankees by turning around in a corner of a cabin. He also realized that they had to defeat one enemy at a given time.

Carberry stated, "Chemung is swarming in Tories as we talk!" "I have seen them with my own eyes!" Three miles from Ester's Town, Shawnee

Village was retaken by us last night. I left my men there, and moved with two other men to a mountain overlooking Chemung. Carberry reported that they are already forming, and at least 200 Indians have gathered there with the Tories of Young Butler.".

Denison asked, "What about the Wyoming Rangers?".

"They are too tired to march and they are around Ester's Town."

Carberry added, "More last night." He shook his head in anticipation of their next question. "The town's abandoned. Ester is on the hoof. Who knows where? I think the scouts are grabbing as much plunder as they can in canoes. There are nearly two dozen canoes. "I left the rest of my men to drive cattle and horses that we've captured and to form an rear guard." He looked at all the men in the eyes. He looked at Colonel Hartley, who was looking deathly into his eyes. "Sir Chemung sir, more than three hundred Tory Rangers there alone with at least two hundred brave savages!" Are you ready to march against us?"

Hartley rubbed his chin and said "My God", "Three hundred? They

They must have thought our numbers were great, or they would have swooped upon us now, for certain. This will be our advantage!" He took his canteen and shook it. He poured a little whiskey into it. "We are nearly out of food and we feel afflicted. Five hundred more men are available to us. We need to get as much sleep as possible today and then collect as many provisions and plunder as we can.

All officers nodded.

Hartley nodded at them. Hartley stared at them with wide eyes.

Something behind the officers caused them to immediately turn around.

From the north, dozens of smoke columns curled into the air. The billowing columns were joined by smaller columns just above the trees. They are black and rolling.

Hartley stated that "The scouts will soon return with their horse," "They've

Put the torch to Ester's Town. I hope that the smoke will convince our enemies that we are going to advance, and Chemung will be given the torch, because it is all dependent upon it. All depends upon it. Let's get to it! For all of the cabins along the river, there are Tories and savages nests. Send your party! Take all you can and burn it!

Chapter Forty-Four

Colonel Hartley looked at the brave, bending down to knees in front of him. He paced backwards and forth with his hands tightly behind him, his eyes never leaving the brave. The colonel or brave spoke, and the rest of the world waited in silence.

The brave one eye did not become swollen from injury.

The white chief's haughty eyes. Although his body was aching from the rough treatment he received from the scouts' hands, he refused to utter a word, groan or even utter any words, refusing them the satisfaction. He thought back to the fearful look on his children and wife's faces when he heard about the Yankees approaching. This is why he ventured so close to the white eyes, while Queen Ester fled to the glen with the others. He had to strike at devils and then return with a scalp to entice the other fighters to fight. The devils had gotten him. He pondered his fate and his heart dropped. He wished that the chief of the white-eyes would draw his pistol to relieve him from his shame. The white-eyes watched him. This is what kind of torture?

Hartley stopped pacing and walked towards the man. Hartley noticed the brave's reddened eye, swelling and large gash on his head. He stepped back and raised his lower lip. He looked at the freed prisoners and waved his hand at him as he examined them. He called "Captain Smith" and said, "See to this man."

Doctor Smith exclaimed, "Man!" "The good colonel

The word is used loosely.

He examined the recently released man and nodded his head.

The doctor left to follow the orders of the colonel.

Smith said, "Well, orders will be orders," slowly rising from his desk.

The brave walked over to him, kneeling. He looked down at the black-painted miscreant and grunted, pushing the man's head to the side to better see the gash in his eye. He grunted once more and put his hands on the jaw of the brave, forcing his mouth to open. He reported, "He still has his tongue Colonel." He can talk," he reported.

Hartley stood full before the brave and said "Yes indeed." He asked Captain Franklin and Covenhoven, "Do you think that he understands English?".

Covenhoven replied, "He's a Delaware. He's probably Ester's band. Wolf clan." "Most of them are proficient in English, which is why they can trade with civilized people." Covenhoven looked at all of the eyes that were circling him, and nodded.

Some people nodded to his question, but the majority stared at him in dismay.

The foe that caused destruction in their lives.

Hartley asked, "How many are around Chemung?".
Defiance stared back at him through one eye.

Hartley stated, "It's best you answer it, my fine fellow.".
Silence again answered him.
Boss Strope stated, "I'll get that painted pig to squeal!"

With his long knife drawn.

Captain Franklin and Colonel Denison immediately took over

he blocked his path and shook their heads.

"What!? !" Boss said. "With all due respect Colonel Denison.

Fine sir, you've said nothing about this entire expedition! Sir, are you willing to give up your rank? They did it! They know how much they have cost me and mine!" He turned to the many people watching him. "You see what they have done to our families through their treachery!"

Denison stated, "Back off. Private." "Colonel Hartley has in

Command of this expedition. You will obey his orders and treat him with respect. Or, damnit, you'll face the lash upon our return to Wyoming!

Boss snarled and looked at his knife. He threw it to the ground.

In front of the brave. It stuck in the earth, just a hair from the knee of the brave.

The brave didn't hesitate to stand tall.

Denison yelled, "Pick up the knife!" Unmoved by Denison's blatant act

defiance.

Boss looked straight into his eyes, then turned away with a huff. Had

The whole world has gone mad! They had forgotten about Wyoming's field! !

All Iroquois should be condemned!

Franklin sat down and picked up the knife.

Denison apologized, bowing slightly before he said "My apologies Colonel."

Stepping back into the circle with the brave.

Hartley moved towards the brave once more. "Tell us about it!"

He said, "It is all I ask." He said, "It's all I ask."

Hartley's brave yelled, "Go Hell!" and threw their ashes on the ground.

feet.

Many soldiers took a step forward only to be stopped by the

colonel.

He said, "We" and sat down on one knee. The brave looked into his eyes. "Come now, speak and you might see your wife or children again this day. I offer peace and extend the white feather for your chiefs. Many soldiers will follow you, and if you speak now you might curtail bloodshed." The soldiers cried out, "Kill the heathen rats!".

"Silence!" Denison ordered.

The air was filled with muffled taunts.

The brave shouted, "You Bostonians are the ones to die today!" "Five

Chemung is home to hundreds of Young Butlers men! You are as brave as the leaves on trees! You go to Chemung You should not come back with hair!"

Hartley replied, "Well, this is what I meant."

The brave said, "You white-eyes fools!" Van Alstyne, come one, warn you! Many brave will lift your hair and knock on your head! "You will die soon," the brave spat again, looking with all the hatred that he could muster at the Rebel colonel. "You Bostonian, Yank-ee chief, die."

Hartley stated, "I" Hartley, "am not from Boston, but from York."

He knelt down and raised his arms to greet Captain Bush. He asked, "Please give me a quill and some parchment." "I'm sure Captain Butler or Brant can read our message and relay it to the Six Nations," he said. He looked back at Brant, who was vainly trying his best to get up.

Each brave soldier was pushed forward by strong hands.

He was infuriated and he retreated, but he continued to struggle vainly against his bonds.

"Just be still, my dear fellow, and we will be with you immediately."

Hartley said this, raising his coattails to sit on a stump of a log. One soldier sat on a plank and two corn mortars to make a desk. Bush laid the parchment on the plank, and gave the colonel a quill. He also held an inkwell in the other hand.

Hartley licked the quill's end with his lips, and then he dipped it in water.

Ink well. He scrawled on the parchment in a hurry for the longest time. Everyone watched intently. Hartley finally raised with a contented grunt and gave the parchment another look before passing it on to Bush. Bush said, "Make a duplicate of this for Council of War." "And be quick about that, sir, if it's possible."

Bush quickly took the stump left by the colonel, and hastily went to

work.

Hartley spoke of "The Six Nations", walking back to the brave

After reading all that he had written, he said, "have murdered many women and children, as well as ruthlessly tortured many prisoner! This treachery is well-known! It is well-known by all! It is not to be denied! It is imperative that the Chemung chiefs listen to each other and have a dialogue about these issues before peace can be restored among our peoples. They must not delay in suing peace. I say to them all their country will be put to torch and feel the cutting blade of justice!" He looked down at the brave. "They must agree that they will parley before the sun sets above yonder hills, or I swear by the oath that all shall be put to fire and sword. Many come after me. They will be here soon. As Ester's Palace was, Chemung will be passed to the torch! If the Tories don't renounce their misguided loyalty to the Crown, no peace will be reached with them! King George is the greatest tyrant in the world. Their farms will also be torched if the Tories continue to follow their misguided ways! These words will determine the fate of the Six Nations, and the Tories." Bush eagerly gave him the parchment with a confident nod. He turned to the two men who were holding the brave and waved them at him. They let go of the brave slowly. They aimed a dozen rifles at the brave, their grim eyes glancing down at the barrels.

The brave looked in shame at the ground and slowly rose.

Hartley asked Hartley, "Are we to behave? My friend?".
He nodded, but did not look up from the ground.

Hartley asked one of the men for permission to remove the thongs that were holding the Indian's wrists. The gesture was understood by both men, who remained steadfast as if they were unaware of it.

Franklin saw the situation and decided to cut the thongs.

The brave crossed his fingers and shook his hands. He lifted his arms.

Before he could move toward Hartley, he took out his hand and wiped away the blood from his eye.

Twelve rifle locks were clicked as a response.

Hartley was still in his arms when the brave stopped but he held on to Hartley's hand.

Hartley gave Hartley the parchment. Hartley gave him the parchment.

The Chief of Chemung Village. Tell him about all that you see. "I tell you more, come with the thunder tree and are as numerous as the tall grass around this place," he said. He then turned and extended his hand towards the vast sea of Indian grass that grew along the riverbank and north of the village. "We are as strong and as strong as the rough grass, just as it resists any wind blowing against it, so will we!" Go! Now!"

He did not even look at him. He lowered his head instead.

Slowly, he stumbled towards the trail that leads through the waving Indian grass. He began to walk steadily through the village and eventually became a trot. His back disappeared over the crest as he walked through the grass.

Hartley was walking towards Denison, who said "Well." Both were standing

The crowd began to disperse, and Denison sat silently. Denison finally asked, "Do you think that your ruse worked?".
Hartley said "I don't know", Denison could barely hear.

hear. "I only saw the Six Nations through the eyes of one brave, as the other was swollen shut with anger. These people are dealt with by you, what do they think?

Denison stated, "I think, sir, you have done a fine job so."

"Far away." He looked at the lingering smoke columns rising in the northern air. "Ester won't be happy. I have to admit that seeing her castle in flames is a good thing, especially for someone who has been so betrayed. They may be afraid this day, but their scouts will see our true numbers on the morrow.

Hartley replied, "Aye," he said. "I think the exact same." He looked around at his surroundings.

Tired soldiers gather plunder around him. "We will fill every canoe we capture and all the packs-horses' backpacks with what we have. Rest shall be given to the torch. We will get as much rest and keep a strong guard before we return to Wyoming via the Susquehanna. It is the best way for the civilians, cattle, horses, plunder and horses to return. After this day, it will be at the long trot every step." He stopped and looked north. "No word from Colonel Morgan's riflemen nor Colonel Butler with Fourth Pennsylvania. I had hoped that I could join them here and accelerate the march so as to meet the enemy around Chemung. But, alas, they haven't deemed it suitable to rendezvous with me. We will, however, continue to march according to our new plan.

Denison stated, "It's a reasonable plan sir." "I concur."

Hartley, gazing at the tall mountains, said "I am glad."

They surround them. "But, you are correct, many eyes will soon gaze down on us from the mountains. Our only hope lies in our little ruse. But if it does come to it, I would give up any of my men to thrice our number."

Denison jerked at the words. They were already familiar to him.

He prayed for a different outcome at the Battle of Wyoming. He said, "I pray that it will not happen to that." But if it does, these men would give them all the pain and suffering they deserve from Wyoming's rape. This is certain.

Hartley stated, "Amen to it." Hartley said, "Amen to it."

Chapter Forty-Five

In the early morning, the Susquehanna was smacked by flames from dozens upon dozens of burning cabins. A small group of canoes sailed silently down the river, breaking it with slight splashes and ripples. The canoes were paddled by three-cornered, round, and wide-brimmed, slouch-hat-wearing Grim Faced Men. They all looked downstream and beyond the twisting mountains.

Mounted men whistled as they herded livestock along the trail.

riverbank. Others, riding horses and heavily armed, galloped along a swathe of civilians and men. In their wake, beams cracked and fell. The horsemen, who were the ones leading the way, took no notice of the destruction they left behind and all but one turned. All eyes were now set on leaving this Indian country in search of safer havens further downstream, namely the Fort at Wyoming.

Captain Bush's musicians did not perform any lively airs for their backs

They were laden with plunder. The preacher at head of the civilians exclaimed "Hallelujah!" with nearly every step down the trail. This was probably because his back didn't have a bundle. He explained that his burden was to safely transport his flock down the river. To accomplish this difficult task, he needed every ounce of his body and soul. His praises for God were not hindered by the bundles he placed on the backs his flock. He explained that the Lord's ways were indeed mysterious to the soldiers.

Colonel Hartley pushed his horse up to the top of the column.

Escape the sermons of the preacher and silently wonder if the man didn't play an act for Indians who were watching from the mountains above. The Indians were afraid of a touchy man and let him do whatever he wanted, so long as they stayed away. He thought that the Lord works in mysterious ways and tried to put the thoughts of the man out his mind so he could focus on the trek ahead. Wyoming lay eighty miles downstream. He wondered how they could survive this stretch of wilderness as dangerous as the Sheshequin Path.

They had no choice but to try, and they did. He was afraid for their fate, which God would decide.

Before the horse rose above the trail, he reined the horse.

steep Narrow Way, and waited for his pack-horse train. He looked down at the still-mumbling preacher, and wished he had practiced silence being gold, especially now. He nodded at Lord Butler as he watched him pass.

Lord nodded, gesturing towards the single sack of flour on his right.

He left behind his pack-horse. Hartley was shocked to discover that there were only a few small whiskey kegs on the pack-horse right after it. All manner of plunder was found wrapped on the horses of the rest of his train. He only wished that the Indians' dogs hadn't been as thorough in consuming the Indians stashes before they skedaddled from their villages. They had done a good job for their masters. Their enemy was repelled by plunder. It was made easier by food.

Lord asked him, "Is that all there is left of the provisions?"

riding up behind him.
Lord replied, "I'm afraid so Colonel", waving towards the

Herd of cattle. "But we have plenty of hoofs, if necessary."

Hartley replied, "Yes, son. I think we have." Hartley said, "But what about drink?"

"Well, we'll just need to trust the Lord for the good."

preacher says and hope he protects the water from putrid fever."

Hartley exclaimed, "Quite," and urged his mount forward. He rode to the

Foot of the trail, contemplating the steep climb up to the Narrow Way. Already, a few fell along the trail's edge. With dread, he looked at the approaching column of cattle and civilians.

He called the nearest officer, "Captain Spalding!".
Spalding marched alongside his men and stepped out of his place.

The colonel is the highest. He said, anticipating the words of his commander, "There's an area just a ways back I believe we can ford with any problem.".
Hartley smiled and said, "Very well." "See it! Turn them

"I fear that an ambuscade is waiting for us on this steep path or worse."

Spalding replied, "Yes sir," and turned away to bark orders.
Spalding said, turning away to bark orders.

The car suddenly stopped. "But, there's Breakneck Hill to the east side, just as steep, it's just a few more miles down."

"But the way is much better after that, Franklin has told me," Hartley said, lifting his eyes to the sun rising over the river. "And besides, our tawny friends shall not expect us that way. It'll throw them off a little, perhaps enough for us to get the hell out of here with our hair."
"Sound reasoning, sir," Spalding said, turning to covey the new orders of march.
"Yes," Hartley said under his breath, "I hope it is only sound enough to work, for I fear we may need all of God's graces to get out of this scrape. I do most certainly indeed!"

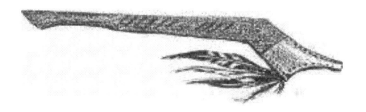

Chapter Forty-Six

Painted men darted from the forest, rifles and spears held ready for action. They dodged in between burning cabins, searching madly all around the ruined village for any lingering white-eyes. But to their disappointment none showed themselves. With sharp hoots they called back to the tree line along the edge of the mountain to the west of the village.

Indians emerged all along the tree line, at first a mere trickle, but soon a flood of miserable and mourning souls. Women wailed upon sight of their burning cabins. Wide-eyed children stumbled about in a daze. All they had known in their entire lives now rose with the thick columns of black smoke billowing in the air. Many cried. Many stood in shock.

One, a middle aged woman, bedecked in bright flashy garments and silver trinkets, stumbled crestfallen to the center of the village. After a while she stopped, staring blankly at a great pile of smoldering ashes lying before her. Collapsing to her knees, she cried a long, slow, mournful wail. Great tears flooded her eyes, flowing down her pale cheeks. She pulled at her long black hair in her grief, flicking her fingers to let strands of it drift in the wind. In no time more women joined her, forming a semicircle around the ashes, the same forlorn wail creeping from all their aching souls.

Warriors stood for a time watching, embarrassed and ashamed no white-eyes paid for this treachery with their blood. Several of them flung their heads back, emitting their own mournful cry. A growing rhythmic thud, slow at first, but increasing with the wails, echoed through the air. At first few eyes turned to see what caused the thud, but with its increasing volume more eyes turned to it, especially the warriors' eyes. The call of war curiously called them forth.

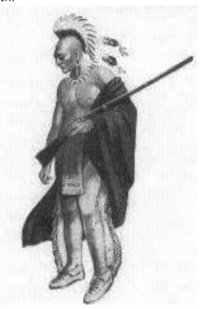

Chief Wamp stood tall beside a slightly charred post, his empty eyes staring straight ahead, seemingly at nothing. His hand rhythmically thudded a red painted post with a war club. More and more warriors crowded around the aged chief. Finally satisfied he drew enough of them, he ceased pounding the post. Slowly, he let the war club fall to his side, his other hand slowly emerging from under the blanket wrapped around his torso. He stretched his arms wide in the air, pushing the blanket from his back. Bright war paint of white, vermillion, and black showed in swirls all over his body.

He lifted his other hand into the air with the war club, yelling in his native tongue. "Brothers! My warriors! Be brave! Be strong! All is not lost!" he called, turning slowly about for all to see his painted body. "I wear the colors of all the wars I have seen! Many battles! Many scalps! The day is not lost!" He pointed the ball of the war club to the sun still low on the horizon. "I say let the woman stay here to mourn! Let the men follow me to meet the white demons before they retreat to Wyoming! Many defiles await them along the trail! We have seen their numbers from the trees! They are no more than ours! The white-eyes of the King say wait! Wait for what? Their escape? I say if Young Butler is too afraid to march when his numbers are so much greater than the devils' then let him stay behind with the women! For that is where he belongs! But all true warriors shall follow me now down the river. The long knives way is long! We know many ways to get ahead of him! He is hindered as always, by his greed! Let us all take up the hatchet and knock him on the head! He is tired! We are strong! He shall pay for his deeds! Come! Brothers! Follow me!"

Another chief, *Panther*, rose in front of Wamp, letting out a horrific yell. He bared his teeth, hissing, his head turning wildly to and fro. His bulging eyes glared into each warrior's soul he encountered. His feet started stomping the ground in a mad rhythm reminiscent of Wamp's thumping of the post. He danced back to the post, smacking it with a sharp whack with his own war club, splintering it into pieces. "This is how we shall strike the white-eyes!" he screamed, collapsing to his knees. Bowing his head, he moaned woefully. His head rose slowly back. His moan rising to a wail, a wail increasing in tone. He jumped at the end of the wail, shaking his body in a spasmodic frenzy of grief. "They have struck our hearts! They have struck our women's hearts! They have struck our children's hearts! Let us strike their dark hearts!"

A medicine man appeared from nowhere and danced around the two chiefs, pulling a reluctant pure-white dog behind him. He jumped and yelled, lifting a flaming firebrand from one of the burning cabins into the air. Two younger warriors hastily threw some wood into a clump before him. He flung the firebrand onto the wood, hissing as the flames grew. With a slow turning hand he waved at the two young warriors. They brought forth three long poles and placed them over the fire, interlocking them at the top.

The medicine man bent down to the dog, cradling the whimpering beast in his arms. Pulling a thick leather thong from his pouch with one hand he looped it around the dog's rear feet. He pulled it tight, tugging and pulling at the thong around the dog's feet, the dog madly trying to crawl away with its fore paws. In one great sweeping arc he lifted the dog by its feet, tying it to the tripod over the fire. The dog whined, jerking furiously against the thong to no avail.

Wamp slowly drew a long knife from his belt and walked up to the struggling dog. His aged but strong fingers reached to the dog's muzzle, clamping it shut while his other hand guided the knife across its neck. Blood flowed copiously down from the flailing dog's neck, sizzling on the fire below it in great spurts with each new spasm of the dog.

The medicine man stood before Wamp and the dying dog and lifted one hand high in the air, with the other flinging gun powder and tobacco onto the sizzling flames. With a high pitched wail, he declared the war sacrifice a success. The great spirit would be pleased and after each warrior partook of a piece of the flesh he would come and make a tobacco pouch of the dog's skin. This the medicine man declared most earnestly.

Panther screamed at the top of his lungs in pure delight. Many warriors joined him.

Wamp stood holding the bloody knife. Gazing at all the enraged eyes beaming back at him he stopped to crack a slight smile when his eyes met another's in particular.

Wamp's wife smiled back at him. Her face still glowed in his memory as it did the first time he ever saw her. He closed his eyes, breathing in the memory, wishing to forever etch it in his mind's eye and silently hoping to recall it if he found himself breathing his last on the battlefield. For he fought for her, their children, and their grandchildren. He fought against the land-crazed and greedy white-eyes. For all they touched turned to ashes.

Ashes whisking in the wind brushed his cheeks. He saw them in his mind, clouding his vision. He forced his eyes against his mind's eye, opening his true eyes to his wife's beaming smile. Taking his knife from his belt he cut the first piece of flesh from the dog. Chewing it slowly he swallowed hard against it. This I do for you, he tried to convey with his eyes to his wife. For you I fight the demons. For you I would die. For all my people I would die.

Wamp's wife recognized the deep stare, as always wondering

what burned in her husband's soul when his eyes glared so. It remained a mystery to her, but she felt fine with it, for some feelings escaped words. She did as she always did at the look, she smiled.

Chapter Forty-Seven

Dark flowed the Susquehanna, dim the haggard souls trudging along its banks. Haunting the light of the pale moon; its glow the only luster in this foreign land. Sullen the eyes staring down to the hard ground from bent heads. Hours ago the sun left them, retreating to its safe haven in the sky. Here they trod, seeking the haven of the fort at Wyoming, but alas, a vast distance lay before them and its safe walls.

No more did the exhausted children walk. Long ago they hitched rides onto soldiers' shoulders. Great bundles of plunder torn from the backs of the pack-horses made a place for their mothers, also, too worn to tread another step.

But onward they must tread; for death followed close behind. No one knew this more than Colonel Hartley. Who but a soldier knows the willing emotions forcing one tired foot after another forward? He raised his nodding head, staring in contempt at the shadows under the great trees surrounding them. He knew they wait there; if not at this very moment, soon. They wanted to kill him. They wanted to kill all who followed his lead. Fighting to open his squinting eyes, he rubbed them again. He felt the large bags under them, thinking he must be an awful sight. Gazing at the haggard souls trudging trance-like around him he knew appearance meant nothing to anyone now. Only life meant something. Only its promise kept them marching.

A bleary-eyed scout stumbled along the line, stopping at the colonel's side. Hartley looked down to him, grunting at him.

The scout nodded and wiped his face with his hand, waving his other forward. His long rifle stood a full foot and a half from the sling on his shoulder; for a second Hartley had the peculiar thought of placing a banner onto it. He shook his head, wiping his burning eyes again. "What is it man?" he growled. "Out with it!"

"The Moravian Indian Village at Wyalusing's just ahead," he

said, pointing at the creek crossing the trail ahead. "That's the Wyalusing Creek just there, once we past it, it's not far at all. Covenhoven says the village's clear, been abandoned some time now, but a few of the cabins survive."   The scout put his arm on the colonel's horse, leaning his tired head against it while he walked. "We all got to rest. Come some thirty miles since Sheshequin. Can go no more, the canoes, all are beached down at the village. Even the paddlers are exhausted."

"Yes, but they've had it much easier than us," Hartley said. "They'll be the guard when we reach the village." He lifted his canteen to his lips, drinking it dry. "Empty," he said. "As is my haversack. We'll have to slaughter a beef at the village and cook up what flour is left into ash cake. From then on we'll live on the beef."

"Fine, sir," the scout said, pushing his head away from the horse's flanks. "I'll push ahead and relay your orders."

"You do that," Hartley said. He never felt so tired. This trek rivaled all he endured with General Arnold in Canada and at Crown Point. Such men, he thought, to endure this without complaint. The preacher complained more than any of his rank and file. Oh, these men. Six Nations beware, for there are legions from where these men came! Attack you bold devils and even in their exhausted state these men shall rip your hearts out of your chests! Yes! These men! He looked to the pale moon, knowing its light also shone on the fort at Wyoming. Somehow he found comfort in the thought. What lack of sleep does to a man's mind! They must rest! They have gained all the ground anyone could through this tangled wilderness. It must have gained them some advantage from their pursuing foe. It must have!

He let his horse ramble down the trail and into the village like the tried souls all around him. He watched men collapse onto the grass. Some kicked in the doors of the cabins still standing, plopping down in exhaustion inside them. Soon an exhausted mass of humanity lay all about the village.

Hartley slid down from the saddle, staggering over to one of the great fires already blazing around the village. He plopped down on the grass beside it and curled into a tight ball, not caring who saw him. The sound of creaking logs being torn from the walls of some of the cabins made him open his eyes for a slight moment. "It's alright," he mumbled. "Tear it all down, burn it all. Raze the whole place so it will be but ashes when we resume the march on the morrow."

No one heard his mumbles over the crackling flames or the bellowing cattle. No one would care anyhow. For survival took over the reins guiding everyone's souls now. Instinct ruled them now, for their enemy hunted them and would probably soon arrive with a vengeance born of hell.

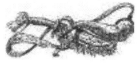

Chapter Forty-Eight

Painted demons, screaming, hollering, and yelling drifted from the forest everywhere, jarring Colonel Hartley awake. His eyes shot open, darting to and fro, the insane vision of his nightmare fading in the light of day. A dream he quickly realized! Just a dream, thank God! His heavy eyelids fell closed again, leaving him somewhere between conscious thought and dreams. But soon the sounds surrounding him; crackling fires, groaning men, baying animals, and sizzling meat over fires, urged him back into reality. He wanted to lie and wait just a few more seconds, perhaps drift back into his uneasy sleep; but alas, the nightmare followed him. He lay with his eyes closed for a few more winks. Thoughts started drifting through the veil of exhaustion clouding his mind.

Here, in the midst of Indian country, sixty miles from the nearest American settlements, with many bands of hostile Indians skulking about their flanks and rear, they sat. The boldness of their movements and the rapidity of their march led their enemy to greatly overestimate their strength. The enemy found no time to rally for defense. But that had changed. Their weakness had been discovered. Hundreds of Butler's Rangers and Johnson's Royal Yorkers had gathered at Chemung alone. Adding Indian forces to their number meant certain annihilation for this small band of courageous men.

Men whom trusted their lives to his leadership, he realized. The weight of the burden kept his eyes closed, but soon he swallowed hard against it, forcing his eyes open to cruel reality.

The haggard and ragged souls tramping around the village brought the full weight of their situation down hard on his shoulders. He sat up, stiffened his back, rubbed his eyes, and rose. Adjusting his hat, he pulled his coat tight at his waist, looking all about.

Few of the exhausted eyes recognized him. The nearest sat around a fire picking at great hunks of beef burdening a great spit over the flames. The smell enticed his senses. He strutted to the spit and drew his knife, cutting a large piece from the chunk of meat. Taking one ravenous bite after another, he swallowed and swallowed until finally the burning sensation in his stomach ceased. Wishing to find anything to wash it down, he reached for a gourd of water sitting by the fire. He took a long drink, noticing the faint bite of whiskey in it.

"We put what whiskey that's left in the water," a soldier by the fire reported to him. "It might take care of the putrid fever within it, leastways, we'll all know soon enough if it didn't."

"Quite," Hartley said, lowering the gourd back down to the ground. "The beef is fine anyhow," he added.

"The scouts slaughtered the best," the soldier said, taking advantage of the rare opportunity to speak freely with one of such high rank. "Fear'n that it might be their last and all, last meal, that is."

"Now see here, my fine fellow," Hartley said, placing one hand on his knee and turning towards the soldier.

The soldier blanched, knowing he had crossed the line with a high ranking officer.

Hartley noticed his fear and shook his head. "Just mind your tongue," he said, "we don't need such talk right now, especially around the poor captives. The thought of returning to captivity among the savages must be most distressing to them to say the least." He nodded his head to one of them he recognized by the fireside. "We will make it to Wyoming," he added, standing tall, "if we have to fight every forsaken inch of the way, we will make it." With that he wandered to the other fires, silently assessing the men's manners and attitudes. All seemed to greet him with confidence and in a self-assured manner; much to his relief. There is always one bad apple, thinking of the brazen soldier who first spoke to him, even in this fine lot. He did not hold it against the man though, for he knew a certain amount of doubt plagued all their minds, no matter what they said.

He drew his watch from his pocket and ignored the admiring looks from all the eyes around him; especially from those of the frontier. For those whom rely on noon marks above a cabin door to tell time, the fancy time piece remained a coveted oddity indeed. Taking out his watch key he wound it, reading its face. "Nearly nine o'clock in the morning," he announced to curious eyes, "we must get ready to march."

Tired heads bobbed in agreement.

"Captain Spalding," he said across the flames. "How are things?"

"Well, sir, most of the men got some shuteye. The ones who were spelled from the watch last night are the ones still resting about. I've ordered all to check their firelocks, for we may have sport today." Spalding answered.

"Very good, Captain, and I am afraid you may be right about sport on this day." He looked to a few mud-caked faces sitting around the fire. Nests of yellow jackets stumbled upon the trail yesterday had done their work. "Has the mud drawn the sting out?" he asked one of them.

"It's helped, but if it ain't that it's someone stumbling over a rut and landing crossways on his tomahawk or the other falling this way or that, twisting their ankles, wrists and such," the man answered.

"Yes, it has been rough going to say the least."

"There are many claiming lameness and some are just done tuckered out," Spalding added to the man's comments. "Many have twisted an ankle and wrist, but no broken bones, as of yet, thank God."

"And how are the men of the regiment?" Hartley asked, turning to Captains Bush and Walker.

"We're holding out fine sir," Walker said. "We got a few stings and twists but we are fit to fight."

"That is fine, for you all," Hartley said. "We shall have to fit what lame souls we can in the canoes and on pack-horses. We have at least two day's march ahead, make sure enough of this beef is boiled for that. Let's get things in order and prepare for the march, I wish to get going as soon as possible. The further we get from Chemung and the closer we get to Wyoming the better I will feel. What say you gentlemen?"

"Huzza to that," the captains said. "Huzza to that, sir."

Chapter Forty-Nine

Colonel Hartley rode up and down the assembling column of his men. Barely one hundred and twenty fell in the line of march, he noticed with a long sigh. Glancing across the green plain to the riverbank, he scratched his head watching the dozens of men filing into the canoes. Some he knew only pretended lameness, but he let them board the canoes just the same. A loud neigh turned his head to the others astride the backs of pack-horses just behind the advance guard of an officer and fifteen men. Several children sat atop oxen, their mothers sitting on pack-horses just behind and to the sides of them. Horned cattle milled about them all, herded by a few of Captain Carberry's Light Horse. The remainder of the Light Horse sat evenly divided between the advance and rear guards.

Hartley stopped, reining his horse about, looking down to the officer in command of the rear guard.

"We'll make it just fine sir," Captain-Lieutenant Sweeney reported to him.

He smiled at the valuable officer and the eager faced lieutenant standing beside him.

"I've five runners, sir," Lieutenant Van Campen said, nodding his head to the men behind him. "Each is as fleet of foot as the next. If we run into mischief you'll know about in a quick hurry, sir."

"Yes, no doubt, Lieutenant," Hartley said, turning an eye to the once fine Indian village, and trying to imagine what it looked like in its heyday, reflecting on the emptiness of war. Many of the cabins, especially the larger ones, sat halfway dismantled. Wide spaces shown between some of the walls. Some fine cedar singles and beams lay scattered about near some of the cabins. They had been torn apart to make timber for rafts, Colonel Denison explained to him, on Lieutenant Colonel Dorrance's late expedition to save the few families up river the previous winter. Now the work would be finished, he thought, waving a hand to the scouts who stood about the buildings with flaming pine knots.

With sharp yells they flung the pine knots into the cabins near them. Grabbing more pine knots from the fire-pits they moved fast and furiously from one end of the village to the other. After they completed their task all of them converged just in front of Hartley. With a satisfied nod from him they scattered to form flanking parties on each side of the column. It had been a beautiful town carved out of the heart of the wilderness by people with no more intention than to live in the peace they preached about from their bibles. Now all the visions of peace went up in flames. They rose with the memory of Wyalusing into the heavens; it's haunting and shadowy memory the only place of peace on this war-torn ground now.

He spurred his horse forward, first riding by Captain Murray's men who formed the Third Division. After saluting them he rode past Captain Spalding's men who formed the Second Division. He also saluted them, before finally taking his place in front of his regiment, which formed the First Division. He looked down to Captain Bush's musicians, nodding his head. Drums promptly beat a strong rhythm of march along with the shrill of three fifes. The spirited music brought new life to the men of the ranks. All stood a little taller.

He glanced down at his watch. Twelve o'clock; noon, as good an hour as any, he thought, casting a defiant gaze up the mountain to their front. The enemy undoubtedly lay in wait for them. How many, he could only imagine, but if they wanted a fight they would get it. With a grim eye and a stiff upper lip, he drew his sword, pointing it to the trail leading up the mountain.

Following the colonel's lead the officer in the advance guard pointed his own sword ahead of him, promptly taking the first step of the march. Every foot behind him stepped in perfect cadence to the beat of the drums, wishing to display their determination to any Indian eyes skulking in the trees somewhere around them.

This little army proved equal to any fight, filled with a terrific resolve pounding in each man's chest. None of their feet would stop marching until they met the gates of Camp Westmoreland, come hell or high water. Damn any Tory, British Regular, or Indian standing in their way. They had come too far and suffered too much for it all to go for not.

A new-born spirit, the *American spirit*, emboldened this new people, born of the old but molded anew by this new land. It forged their hands, their lives, and their spirits. The world never witnessed their spirit before and it frustrated description even in those hearts in which it beat so strongly, but nonetheless it lived, and would live as long as they did, changing their hearts and their descendants' hearts forever.

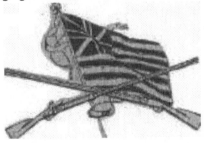

Chapter Fifty

Columns of smoke billowed into the air from the plain behind them. Dark shadows within the great forest lay ahead of them along the lonely trail. None turned to look back, save the rear guard, but faced forward with grim faces full of resolve. Onward to the music they marched, stepping lively with some even singing in the face of the unknown.

Then, as the hornet strikes sudden and quick, flashes of fire erupted in the faces of the advance guard. The flankers yelled, opening a scattering fire. Indian war whoops answered their call. Captain Stoddert calmly ordered the advance guard to 'present' and a breath latter ordered 'fire!' A wall of fire burst from the line of the advance troops. Leaves fluttered. Branches cracked in the thick brush ahead of them.

Colonel Hartley sat resolutely on his mount in front of his regiment, totally confident in Captain Stoddert's ability to handle the threat. If he called for assistance it would be sent posthaste; if not, he could continue on his own.

The anxious eyes of the rank and file did not share their commander's appraisal of the situation. Heads bent around the column, straining to see the fight atop the mountain ahead of them.

"Just keep your places," Hartley called to them. "Watch the flanks and if need be we shall advance!"

Everyone watched puffs of blueish white smoke drifting through the leaves, their perked ears listening to hoots and hollers in the dark folds of the forest. The preacher, overcome with grief, dropped down from an oxen and knelt with a bowed head, beseeching all of heaven to come to their aid.

"Just mind yourself, preacher," Hartley said to him. "Save your request for heavenly assistance for later, for we may need it more then. I suspect this is just a ruse to draw us into an ambuscade. Some of us have learned from Oriskany." He stopped, gazing back to the Second Division. "And Wyoming, I might add."

"We've learned enough to give 'em hell in their own land!" a voice boomed from the ranks.

"Save your spirit, man," Hartley called back to him. "You may find greater need of it before this day is done!"

A wild ball whizzed through the trees to the left of the column, leaving a trail of fluttering leaves in its wake. Women screamed from atop pack-horses and oxen. Wide-eyed children stared in awe of it all, some looking to the staunch colonel sitting resolutely on his horse without flinching.

"All is fine, my dear souls," Hartley assured them with a nod. "Just be still and this shall pass." He barely stopped uttering the words before all fell silent to their front. A faint Indian war whoop sounded in the distance. After it silence prevailed.

A man ran pell-mell from the front of the column, suddenly stopping dead in front of Hartley. "Captain Stoddert's compliments, sir," he reported. "We put the runs to them, sir, Captain Stoddert wishes to know if he should pursue them?"

"No, certainly not," Hartley said. "If they wish to run about and play their games let them, for we are wise to their tricks. We are not following the rascals into an ambuscade. Tell Stoddert to mind the casualties and continue forward!"

"We've no casualties, sir, not even a hair on any of our heads," the runner reported. "The scouts are looking to see if we put a ball in any of them as we speak."

"Tell them to proceed no further and to resume their flanking duties," Hartley said.

"Yes sir!" the runner said, lifting his musket in a hurried salute before scampering up the trail.

"They'll strike again," Colonel Denison said, riding up to Hartley. "They'll strike from ambush and when it's least expected like the snakes they are."

"Yes, Colonel," Hartley said, "but we have a remedy for snake bite! It's swan shot, buck and ball."

"Quite a remedy," Denison said.

"Oh, I think it quite effective, I bet more than a few of the rats in that fight are dealing with stinging lead in their backsides as we speak."

"I hope so, Colonel, I hope so."

"I know so, my friend, I know so."

Both let a slight smile creep across their faces at the thought, quickly erasing it at the sight of the curious eyes of the ranks passing them.

"But it's not over yet, Colonel," Hartley added. "It's certainly not over yet."

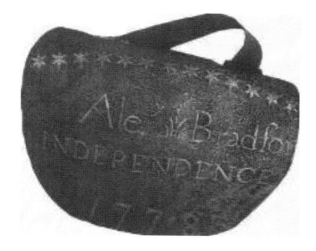

Chapter Fifty-One

The sun climbed high into the sky and turned hot, seeming to awaken every insect and other pest for one last forte. Gnats rose in droves, hovering in clusters around the heads of man and beast. Ticks dropped from trailside brush, growing fat from the blood of many an unwilling host. And always the greatest threat, Indians lurking in the deep shadows of the ever-present forest, plagued everyone's thoughts. They already flitted about their front and stung once, now all hoped their swat good enough to keep them at bay.

Colonel Hartley fanned his hand through a sea of gnats plaguing his face. Annoyingly, they flit about his eyes, seeking its moisture. He ran a finger into the corner of his eye to clear it of their foul presence. He rolled them along his cheek and flicked his fingers, just in time to open his eyes to a new swarm. "My God," he muttered under his breath, "is every pest of the world here today? Indian and insect!'" He almost wished for torrential rains to burst forth from the heavens again but his wrinkled and cracked feet beseeched him to reconsider his wish. He wondered if his feet would ever heal. Part of the rigors of campaigning, he consoled himself, knowing this march may be the axis on which his life turned one way or the other. Fortune or famine lay in it for him and all his troops, he feared.

His eyes fell to one of the scouts kneeling by the trailside, dumping water onto a bare patch of dirt and swirling it about, making mud. He promptly smeared it all over the backs of his exposed hands and neck. "Damn Poison Ivy," he said, noticing the colonel. He angrily waved towards the shiny leaves growing all along the left side of the trail. They stretched and crawled all over the limbs of many of the trees. Falling pine needles and leafs caught in the tangle of ivy vines formed weird and heavy shapes. The matting of vines stretched as far as the eye could see into the forest, giving the trees a strange appearance of some new form of threatening beasts rising from hell itself.

"You flankers do your best," Hartley said, noting the difficulty of the ground and their fatigue. "It is all I ask of any of you." Another cry from the line made him and everyone else look to men in the ranks slapping at their bodies.

Another nest of yellow jackets must have been disturbed. All of this, Hartley cursed under his breath, with an enemy posed to strike at any moment. It seemed the children of the forest had entreated their Gods for help and they had responded by causing every manner of pest to descend and plague their foes.

Slapping at a bite on the nape of his neck he turned his open hand. staring at a great glob of black flesh mushed into it. My God, now horseflies joined the assault. He felt his horse's tail flail against its rear flanks. Its loud neighs of frustration echoed along the trail. But the sound echoed alone, save those recently stung, for not a grumble sounded from the troops plodding along beside him. "Such men," he said on a sigh. "Such men." He swallowed hard against his parched throat. Another problem of which he heard no complaint, thirst. Even though they marched on full bellies of beef few drank the only thing left to them, water, for fear of 'putrid fever'. Some had mixed what little whiskey remained in their canteens with the water, hoping to stave off putrid fever, but most declined to drink it. Thirsty, tired men, but not a murmur of complaint rose from their dry throats. "Such men," he whispered again, wiping sweat from his eyes. Sixty miles to go, his scouts told him repeatedly. Sixty miles of hell. He thought of the men in the canoes, envying them. "We must push on," he muttered under his breath. A few eyes in the ranks looked to him. "We must push on," he said louder, hoping to ease their apparent concerns. "Push on! We need all good men to their duty just now! The enemy is all around! We must keep on! Keep a sharp eye and a sure foot!""

Just then a man stumbling just to his rear fell, rolling down the edge of the steep trail. He quickly rose to his feet, searching madly for his fallen musket and hat. In his exhausted state he barely noticed the odd angle of his tomahawk stuck in his belt, and the growing red spot around the head of the weapon. Finally noticing it, his eyes bulged. Amazed, he dropped both hat and musket, grabbing at the tomahawk and carefully pulling it from his thigh. "Just a scratch," he reassured himself. "It's just a scratch!"

"Here now," a sergeant called down to him. "Be still, I'll be down directly to help." The sharp crack of dozens of rifles stopped the sergeant dead in his tracks. He lifted his own weapon, listening. Another volley, followed by war whoops and sporadic rifle shots, echoed through the air. The sergeant hurriedly met the wounded man and helped him back to the ranks, all the while being assured by him of his need for no aid. "Just a scratch," the man countered the sergeant's concerned look at his wound. In no time both took their place in the ranks, paying little heed to the 'scratch'.

"Form up!" Hartley called to the troops, drawing his sword. "We shall make short work of them!" He spurred his mount up to the crest of the trail, quickly surveying the ground. A slight ridge rose above a swale from which puffs of white smoke ascended in the air.

He cast an eye to Captain Stoddert busily ordering his troops forward in good order along with some scouts. "Good job, Stoddert," he said under his breath. "Keep them busy and we shall flank them." Trusting in the competent officer to keep the enemy engaged, he rode back to his awaiting troops, reassuring the nervous preacher, women, and children while he rode through their number.

"Second and Third Division!" he called to the awaiting troops. "Move to the left and flank the enemy! First Division form on me!"

Captains Spalding and Murray instantly barked out commands to their troops. Both led their troops up the left side of the trail and into the woods fearlessly, ordering those with bayonets to fix them on the march. Their backs quickly disappeared in the woods.

Hartley and the others stared into the depths of the forest swallowing them up, anxiously awaiting any sign of their progress. "You men form up right here," he ordered his regiment. "Fix bayonets! Refuse the flank, while the rest face forwards. We don't know from which direction the devils may strike, we must be prepared!"

A sharp volley, followed by another, broke the haphazard sound of musketry. Soon great yells of triumph sounded from the woods, To Hartley's relief in English.

"They've broken them," Hartley said, perking up in his saddle, listening intently. No war whoops or spurts of rifle fire echoed through the air. A slight rustle to their left caused an awful moment of concern before triumphant brown-coated men appeared from the woods, followed by others in a wide array of civilian and military dress. Spalding marched proudly in their lead with Murray by his side, a self-satisfied grin stretching across both of the officers' faces.

"We put them to their heels for sure, sir," Spalding reported. "They'll be thinking about our little surprise all the way back to Chemung."

"Oh, I only wish," Hartley said. "But me thinks they are about some other mischief. We, my good man, may have a sharper encounter before this is all done."

"Perhaps we should seek them out," Murray said.

"Where?" Hartley asked, rolling his eyes to the thick forest. "They could be anywhere, and we have civilians, cattle and such to mind. No, it is best we be on our way with what we have, trusting in providence to deliver us from this hell."

"Amen! Colonel, amen!" the preacher exclaimed, overhearing his words.

"Quite," Hartley said with a nod to the nervous man of the cloth. "This was only an amusement on their part, though your movement did put a cork in their bottle of mischief, for sure. Good job, very good job, for you all!"

Lowering his voice to Spalding he asked "Do you think you inflicted any losses on the enemy?"

"Hard to tell, sir," Spalding said, "the way they scatter and carry away their dead and wounded."

"Yes," Hartley said, nodding his head to Stoddert's runner approaching them. "Are there any casualties of Stoddert's men?" he asked the man before he reported.

"No sir," the runner answered. "It was getting a little hot when the Captain Stoddert said to hold fast and you would send a surprise into their flanks, then, pop! there was these men spilling out the woods! The enemy scattered like the wind! Sir! Like the wind!"

"Very well," Hartley said. "Give Captain Stoddert my compliments and tell him to resume the march at once. We had one man slightly wounded in an accident, but we are all well, and shall follow with all due haste. We must lose as little time as possible with the enemy. Perhaps in this we shall foil any of his attempts of ambuscade. So let's get to it!"

Chapter Fifty-Two

Hawkins Boone stopped his paddle in mid-stroke, perking his head towards the shore. The man in the rear of the canoe, John Brady, compensated for the drifting canoe with quick strokes from his paddle, staring at Boone in wonder. What did he sense? These Boones, all of them he heard tell of anyway, possessed a sixth-sense about things. None had a keener sense than Hawkins, though, besides maybe his cousin Daniel in the Kentuck country. Brady lifted the edge of his paddle out of the water, straining an ear to listened for what alerted his friend's senses. Those in the canoes behind them also noticed Hawkins, lifting their paddles from the water.

Silence drifted over the swirling face of the Susquehanna. No one moved in the drifting canoes except one or two bending down to their rifles. Hawkins slowly lifted his hat from his head, waving to the others behind him.

He kept his head bent towards the riverbank, intently listening to something none of the others heard.

John Brady scanned the shore, his hand falling to the pistol in his belt. He still didn't hear or see anything out of the ordinary, but he trusted his friend's senses. Several sharp cracks from the mountain on the east side of the river caught his attention. He leaned his head towards the noises. The further they drifted the louder and sharper the cracks sounded, joined by the faint cry of yelling men and the unmistakable cries of the rage of war. Everyone sat rigid in the canoes, anxiously waiting for the sounds to increase or die as the previous noises had but a half hour before these shots.

They increased.

Hawkins Boone immediately sank his paddle deep into the river, paddling madly for the riverbank. Brady followed his lead, along with everyone else. Soon all the canoes sat beached silently on the muddy riverbank. No one spoke, but reached for their rifles and accoutrements.

Listening to the sounds of battle rising on the mountain before them, they formed into a long line, suddenly relieved or forgetting about their so-called ailments.

All eyes ran up the line to Boone, who stood listening and staring up the mountain. He looked to Brady before turning to William King. Both men nodded at him. He nodded back, pointing forward with his rifle. The whole line instantly started up the mountainside, moving silently and gracefully as to put to shame any pack of wolves. All focused on the sounds of battle ahead and negotiated the terrain in perfect unison, leaving no one but two guards for the canoes behind, or anyone exposed to their front. They moved as one.

The abating sounds of battle did little to break their tight formation. Each a seasoned woodsman, they knew the importance of keeping together against the fury of their foe. Experience taught them to stand fast at the first shock; after which the Indians seemed to lose face and melt away into the forest. They seemed to have little stomach for a stand up fight one on one, at least from their experiences with them, of course with the exceptions of Oriskany and Wyoming. The exceptions played hell with their reasoning, but onward they marched.

A growing silence blanketed the mountain. Moving carefully as not to disturb the silence, they broke the crest of the trail, fanning out in every direction. Some carefully examined the trailside, while others combed over the apparent scene of battle.

Hawkins Boone himself seemed to be everywhere at once, by the trailside, front and rear, and to the battlefield itself. He finally stopped, running a careful eye over a slight clearing to their front. Bits of paper from torn cartridges lay strewn all over the area, along with the other litter of every battlefield, bits of torn leather straps, neglected haversacks, a couple of hats, a stray buckle or two, and even a powder horn.

"They beat feet in a hurry," Brady said, scanning the clearing beside Boone. "But there ain't no sign of anybody hurt, thank God. From the looks of things they can't be far up the trail."

"Yep," Boone said. "They did beat feet in a hurry, rightly so, for the Copperheads are merely playing with them, slowing them to strike them at some spot they choose better up the way." Squinting his eyes, he looked up the trail. "Colonel Hartley's right smart about it. He knows the foxes are circling the hen house. Thinks it's best to just keep moving as fast as he can, leastways he might spoil a bit of their sport and get away from them afore they's ready."

Brady nodded in conformation and to the others forming around them. "Ambush, as always," he said.

Hawkins nodded.

"There ain't no one about these parts, white or red," a gruff looking man in buckskin reported to him. "They's all gone down the trail."

"Over here!" a man called from back down the trailside. They all scampered down the trail, looking down to the man.

The man waved at some disturbed dirt and bushes, his hand flowing down to ground at his feet. Kneeling down he raised a few leaves up in his free hand. Holding the leaves to his face, he smelled them, then tasted something on the leaves. "Blood," he said, lowering the leaves, letting them dance in the breeze down to the ground. He lifted his rifle, looking all about the mountain. "It's people blood, too, ain't no horse or varmint, excepting maybe an Injun, but by its place it looks like someone was shot, fell, or was pushed down the bank and ended up here. Ain't no blood trail after this spot, so I reckon he got the bleeding stopped."

"Well, they've drawn blood," William King said. "Once they get the taste of it there's no stopping them, the snakes."

"Could have been someone just fell," Brady said.

"Was you a hearin' the same ruckus we was a coming up here?" King asked, shaking his head and pointing to a small sapling cut in twain by a ball just a few feet from them. "With all that lead flying it's a miracle if no one caught a ball, white or red, Tory or Patriot!"

"That may be," Boone said, looking down the mountainside to the river. "But we best get back to them canoes and get to paddling downriver to keep astride with them. I have an awful hankering that the colonel just may need a miracle afore this day is done, for I fear many a tomahawk may be about his head! And he might just get a miracle from canoes on the river. So let's get to it!"

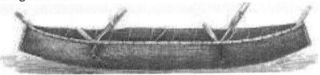

Chapter Fifty-Three

The tight trail led into a thick marsh, made all the worse by the recent rains, but onward they trod. Stunted trees stood about the gnarled swamp. Lichencovered rocks lay above the mucky water. Slimy blue-green algae covered the tree trunks in the morass. The mucky water smelled of rotting plants and soggy earth. Men's and horses' feet made a strange sucking sound with each step. All eyes stared to the other end of the trail and the promise of solid footing. The trees ahead seemed less dense and the ground rose slightly, showing hints of a rocky face. All wondered why on earth the trail cut through the swamp, but after looking to the sheer bank to the right cascading down to the river and the slight rill of water running through a tangle of vines and stumps along with trees covered with poison ivy to the left, the wonder escaped them. They bowed their heads, plunging along the soggy trail.

Hartley plopped down from the back of his struggling horse, sinking knee deep in the muck. Grunting in disgust, he braced himself against the flanks of his horse, pulling one foot, then the other, from the thick mud. Besides a few eyes glancing his way, no one offered him any help.

They had their own troubles.

Laying his arms across his horse he took a few deep breaths. Watching Carberry lead his exhausted mount along the trail in front of him, he wondered of their effectiveness if trouble awaited them further up the trail. But they all ached and longed for sleep. The Light Horse behaved magnificently so far, and he scolded himself for his doubts about them.

The caw of several crows over the trees ahead of them rolled his tired eyes towards them. They flew towards them, then suddenly turned towards the river after catching sight of the haggard line of people, cattle, and horses struggling through the swamp. Even Hartley drew something of the fact they did not fly in the direction from which they originally took to the wing.

"Something has spooked them," Captain Murray said, trudging through the muddy water just to his side. "It'll be our friends calling upon us again, probably in those trees just ahead or there about. Trees aren't so thick there, but just enough to give some cover while firing on us on the trail below them." He lifted his rifle barrel towards the trees. "Bet my life on it, I would, yes sir."

Hartley watched the crows, digesting the passing captain's words. No doubt they had merit, for Murray had a great knowledge of Indians and the same strange sixth-sense Hawkins Boone possessed. He nodded to Murray's men marching behind him. All of them perked their heads towards the crows, each pondering their warning.

Hartley's mind flashed with scenarios of battle. Mr. Stoddert, stern, competent, and professional, along with his mixture of riflemen, scouts, and militia, would be fine. Mr. Sweeney, just as capable, would be fine in the rear. If need be he would dispatch Captain Spalding and his hardy men to their aid. Each a fine shot, they could hold against thrice their number. He could divide Mr. Murray's men wherever needed along with the Light Horse. That left only the center with the cattle, civilians, pack-horses, and his regiment. Fine in proper line of battle against a red-coated and proper foe facing them, his men proved awkward at woods fighting. But with swan shot in each musket they would prove just as valuable. He liked Captain Spalding's idea of sequential fire, a necessity in fighting Indians who waited for their enemy to fire and then rushed them before they could load again.

Watching the men march past, another thought burdened his mind. His responsibility for their wellbeing played hard at his conscience. He tried to rationalize it away, but it plagued him just the same. Here, if one fell, fifty miles from any help, he lay at the mercy of the land and savage; both of them as unforgiving and ruthless as the other. He must do his best, he told himself: For these men, and for himself. He rubbed his eyes, reassuring himself of his plan before stepping through the muck again.

After trudging for what seemed hundred miles through the muck, he sighed in relief upon touching solid earth again. With his first step he stumbled over one of the many rocks, finding himself cursing it. He pulled angrily at the reins of his horse but then let up on them, curbing his anger with his resolve. One must not lose his bearing, he told himself, especially when tested in such an inhospitable place. He looked through the trees surrounding them. The ground stretched and rolled gently underneath great, towering branches of ancient trees. It all took on the appearance of a fine park, no doubt from the custom of the Indians burning the scrub brush away under the trees by controlled fires, he reasoned. He had heard of the practice, but now witnessing its effect he admired it. No wonder the Indians fought so hard in their own country.

The rolling ground crested over a ridge just ahead, beyond it a spectacular view of green rolling mountains stretched under the deep blue sky. Such beauty, he thought, could only be inspired by the hand of the divine. All of the sudden the gnats and black flies seemed frivolous compared to the majesty of this place. Now he knew why the Wyoming people cherished this land so much. It must be fought for. It must be won.

The sharp crack of rifled guns rudely broke him out of his trance. He looked to his front. Seeing nothing, he realized the sounds came from the rear. He turned his horse aside and quickly mounted it, yanking its reins towards the sound of the new battle. Hundreds, not dozens as before, of shots echoed through the air. He spurred his horse to Captain Spalding, immediately ordering, "Second Division to the rear!"

Spalding and his men sprang to the task, marching at the long trot to the rear. One of Van Campen's runners hurried past them with a look of horror in his eyes. Ignoring him with the calm of a soldier's eye, stern and grim, they ran steadfastly to the sound of battle. Duty called!

"They are in force, sir!" the runner reported to Hartley.

"Yes, I can hear," Hartley said. "I am sending the entire Second Division to your support, tell Sweeney to hold fast!"

"Yes, sir," the runner said, turning to catch up with Spalding's men. Screeches he never heard before, produced by fiends he thought only imaginable in his grimmest nightmares, turned his head to the left of the line. A burst of murderous fire flashed from the trees all along the left, felling several surprised men in Hartley's front.

"Stand fast!" Hartley bellowed, yanking his sword from its sheath. Quickly raising it, he defiantly pointed it towards the trees. "Form on me!"

The men of his regiment dutifully obeyed, ignoring the men writhing in pain to their front. They formed a smart line, standing rigidly and firm.

"Make ready!" Hartley screamed. The whole line of firelocks flew from the shoulder to their front. "Present!" The firelocks leveled. Hammers clicked back. "Fire!" A wall of lead splattered against the trees, splintering saplings and thudding hard into branches and trunks. Teardrop shaped swan shot flittered through the leaves. Several groans sounded in the wake of the horrific volley, despite of the Indians ducking when they heard the colonel's orders.

"Captain Bush!" Hartley said, "Independent fire, but keep it sequential, one fire while the other loads!"

A new chorus of gunfire caught his ear from the front of the column. Glancing down at Bush, he spurred his horse toward the new sounds. "Third Division follow me!" he said to the anxious men left standing behind the line of his regiment.

Stoddert stood full in front of his men, pointing his sword with one hand at painted men skulking in the bushes to their front while firing his pistol with his other hand. A half dozen of his men slowly advanced against the enemy with their officer, laying down a constant and steady fire.

Only Stoddert turned to look out of the corner of his eye to Hartley galloping hard from the rear to them. "We have them well in hand here, sir," he reported over his shoulder. "We'll put the run to them shortly!"

Hartley glanced madly about, taking in all of the characteristics of the land. "They are pushing from the rear," he said to Murray. "Look to that ridge! If we gain it, we can pour a broadside into them!" "Yes, sir," Murray said.

Just before he finished speaking a runner from the rear, Van Campen himself, rushed up to him. "Colonel! They are driving us from the rear!" he reported. "We're holding, but it's getting hot!"

"Damn it but for those men in the canoes!" Hartley said, staring down towards the river. "Look at the lay of the land! But for a few more men we could completely surround them!"

"Surround them hell, sir, with all due respect," Van Campen said. "They're doing just that in our rear!"

A horrible shrill echoed through the air. Great blue-white clouds of stagnant smoke hung lazily about the ridge. The acrid smell of sulfur quickly filled the air, hanging low in the stagnant and humid air, burning eyes and choking men. Indians yelled from all quarters. White warriors screamed just as loudly back at them. Curses, taunts, and threats screamed forth in a dozen different tongues. Women screamed with fright from atop jittery packhorses and oxen. Hearty prayers sounded between their yells from the terrified preacher. The Light Horse dashed in and about the trees on their exhausted and played-out horses, screaming and firing their weapons while brandishing their long sabers at the scattering foe darting in and among them. Men fell from horses and onto the ground all around, some painted, some in blue regimentals, some in buckskin, and some in breech-cloths.

The chaos of battle spread out everywhere before Hartley's eyes. He thought of his promise to himself and to his men. If anyone fell, he knew no quarter would be given, on both sides.

Watching two of Stoddert's men wrestle a huge brave to the ground and dash his brains out of his skull bore witness to that fact. The gleam of a knife shone in the chaos and smoke. He watched it slice the scalp lock from the fallen brave's crown with one quick flick of a wrist. Before the two men rose from their gruesome task, spears and arrows rained down on them, one screaming "powder and ball doth settle all!" and kneeling, firing his rifle. The other stopped dead in his tracks for a heartbeat. He turned towards Hartley, his eyes pinched together staring at a long rod protruding from his forehead. Before raising his hand to it a gush of blood poured down from the arrow, flooding his eyes. His body going limp, he fell instantly to the ground.

No more would he breathe, Hartley thought just as a glancing blow from a feathered lance struck across his horse's shins. It jumped, nearly throwing him from its back. He gripped its mane, steadying it by leaning forward and whispering in its ear. A shadow of a breeze passed his cheek followed by a whizzing sound. He brushed at his cheek and drew his pistol, firing at painted men darting between the trees to his side. "Pour it into them!" he screamed, joining his men in cursing the awful savages. "Send them all to hell this day! Send them to hell, dear boys, to hell!"

He watched his regiment fight the painted men darting about their

front. Standing firm, they fired briskly, matching the rate of fire from their foe fighting from behind trees. Several enemy balls peppered their ranks. Men screamed, twisted and fell in agony, spilling blood in great spurts onto the ground and one another. A few broke from the ranks, charging independently at shadows in the smoke and trees, some emerging victorious, others falling from a hail of angry lead.

"Stand fast!" Hartley screamed. "Don't let them drive you in! Stand fast and fire! Dear boys, stand fast and fire!"

Obeying, none ventured forth after hearing their colonel's order. Soon the bursts of flames from the trees lessened, and the yells sounded from behind, instead of their front.

"We've got to gain the ridge!" Hartley said. "They're concentrating on our rear!"

"Permission to flank, sir!" Stoddert asked, waving his sword to the opposite side of the ridge.

"Do as you see fit, man, but keep your hair, mind you!" Hartley said, turning his horse towards the mass of men scrambling to gain the ridge. Arrows, bullets, and spears peppered them but they plod headlong to the ridge, knowing their very survival relied on following orders.

"I intend to keep my hair, but may lift a few of the Indians' locks!" Stoddert answered, leading a dozen men into the trees he so recently freed of their foe.

"Godspeed," Hartley called behind them. "Godspeed!" He quickly loaded his pistols and stared at the ridge ahead, hoping and praying he and his men reached it before the enemy realized their designs. "Rush on boys! Rush on!"

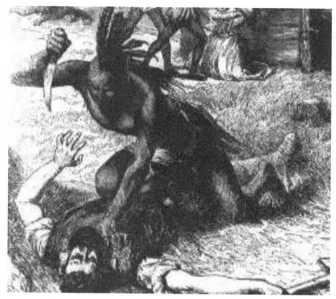

Chapter Fifty-Four

Captain Spalding stood tall at the apex of his line of men, directing their fire and calmly reassuring them. Balls whizzed all about the line, striking the ground and thudding into the trees around them. "Keep it hot!" Spalding called to his men, "pour it into them! Hold them, damn it! Hold them!" He rolled his eyes to his left. Sweeney and his men stood firm, but a new rain of fire struck them, knocking several to the ground.

With loud yells and bulging eyes a group of Indians burst headlong into Sweeney's staggering line. Soon more poured one after another into the line. Rifles swung in the air at them, along with tomahawks, swords, and fists. Men of both sides fell, rolling to the ground in masses of flailing arms and legs. Screams and oaths in many tongues sounded from the smoky ground.

In the midst of the mayhem a slight tug at his arm twisted Spalding about. Glancing down at his shoulder he noticed a fresh tear in his brown regimental. He grabbed at it and pulled it up, to his relief finding no blood spewing from the tear. He looked to his right, seeing white men in green hunting shirts madly reloading their weapons and firing into his line. "To the right oblique!" he ordered his line. "Take aim! Fire!" A dozen firelocks fired in unison into the brush to his right, delivering a hail of fire. One of the green-shirted men twirled about, clutching his arm. Others grabbed him, dragging him along in hasty retreat.

Spalding glared at them. Madly reloading his pistol, he called "Elliot! Terry!" to the two men nearest him in the line. "Scout the to the right. Make sure no more Tory rats are lurking there. Clear it if you can! Clear out the rats!"

Joseph Elliot and Jonathan Terry instantly backed from the line, dashing to the right. Spalding watched them disappear and called to his lieutenant, "Jenkins hold them here! I've got to see Sweeney!"

Jenkins nodded. With grim eyes, he calmly loaded his rifle. Raising it, he took careful aim at two of the painted men dashing from the trees towards Sweeney's men on his left. He fired. One of the braves tumbled and rolled on the ground, only to be quickly dragged back into the trees by his comrade.

Spalding nodded, praising the great shot with a wide grin. A spear flying from nowhere wiped his grin away. He flinched just at the right moment, watching the spear thud into the ground between his feet. He swiped it with his sword in anger, cutting it in twain. Lifting his pistol in his other hand he fired at numerous miscreants hiding behind the trees. "It's getting hot," he said to Covenhoven, noticing the awe in his eyes from witnessing the whole spear episode. "You want to come with me to Sweeney? We've got to coordinate our actions. They're concentrating on us, and I've seen some Tory rats sulking about!"

Covenhoven fired once more ahead of him and scampered over to the captain, reloading while he ran. Both men strode through the arrows, bullets, and spears flying and striking all around them. Smoke engulfed the entire line, trees and all, and both looked apprehensively at the screaming braves darting about the smoke and trees.

Sweeney barely lifted his eyes from his front to acknowledge the officer's and scout's approach when a new wave of warriors burst forth, striking his line with all their fury. The crack of several men's skulls attested to their rage.

A large warrior strode through the smoke directly at Sweeney, sweeping the men's clubbed rifles aside with ease. 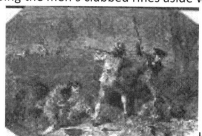 He gripped a tomahawk in his white knuckles, raising it high over his head to strike.

Sweeney's pistol clicked. No fire spurt from it to check the advancing demon of death. Instantly he raised his sword and spun about, deflecting the blow of the tomahawk enough so it just skimmed his cheek. Sinking down, he twirled about on his right foot.

In the same moment the brave raised the tomahawk again, baring his teeth at the Rebel officer. He drew his knife from his belt, raising it in his other hand.

Sweeney's sword, riding on the momentum of his twirl, struck up and into the brave's ribcage.

The brave's eyes widened in shock. He cocked his head to one side, dropping both tomahawk and knife. His hands fell to the sword, grabbing it to no avail, blood flowing from his palms from his grip on the blade.

Sweeney raised one foot to the brave's thigh, slowly drawing the blade out of his ribcage. A great spurt of blood sprayed forth on the brave's last gasp. His eyes rolling back in his head, he fell hard on top of his slayer.

Both Spalding and Covenhoven rushed to Sweeney, gruffly pulling the dead brave off their exasperated comrade.

He quickly rose, covered with smudges of vermillion paint and peppered with blood. Furiously wiping the blood from his eyes with his sleeve he greeted the officer and scout. "My God! They're pouring all they have into us! They're mad! They're insane!"

"Yes, mad with fight!" Spalding said, his eyes widening in awe of a new wave of red men charging from the trees through the smoke. He raised his pistol and Covenhoven his rifle. Both fired at the same instant, felling the same brave.

Sweeney turned around, quickly picking up his pistol. Aiming at an aged warrior in the forefront of the Indians he pulled the trigger. This time it sparked to life, but in his haste Sweeney jerked the weapon to his left. The ball creased the warrior's skull to the aged chief's right. The warrior fell backwards, screaming and clutching both of his hands to his head. Suddenly rising, he ran pell-mell back to the safety of the trees.

The aged warrior glanced back at him and turned about, his eyes full of purpose and anger. He screamed something in his native tongue so loudly it rose above the mingled roar of battle. He darted forward, carrying a dozen or more warriors in his wake. Smoke swirled about his grisly painted body by the sheer force of his mad steps. He swung his war club savagely to his right and left, clearing a huge swath of Rebels before an equally angry volley felled several of the warriors following him. With great reluctance, he turned and retreated back to the trees, cursing the white demons.

Covenhoven fired into them and lowered his rifle to reload it. His eyes wide, he turned to the two officers standing next to him. "That chief said *'My brave warriors we drive them; be bold and strong, the day is ours!'*" he reported.

"Damn it, the bloody savage, I'll give him a day he'll regret!" Spalding said. Reloading his pistol, he backed with the line being pushed by a renewed burst of brisk fire. He fired along with the rest in the line and looked to his own line holding strong on the right. Before long his men stumbled back until they fell out of his view, forming a gap in the line.

A new, somehow more furious wave of painted men darted

forward, plowing into Sweeny's staggering line. Men met hand to hand in mortal combat. Several swarmed around Spalding. A long spear thudded into a man at his side. The man fell to his knees, cursing all of heaven and hell.

His foe darted towards him, ready to finish his work with his upraised tomahawk. Spalding leveled his pistol at him when a spine-tingling wail to his front instinctively turned his pistol to a crazed man bearing down on him. He fired, killing the man within an angry step of him. Looking in the same blinking of his eye he watched Sweeney's man grasp and yank the spear from his bowels, gasping and twisting it in the same instant to meet an advancing demon to his own front.

The brave's momentum sank the spear clean through his bowels, popping it out his back. Instinctively, he reached forward, clutching the wideeyed white man before him by his shoulders him in his death grip.

The white man's hands gripped the spear impaling his foe with his own death grip. Blood spilled from of the corners of his mouth along with many gurgled curses.

Both men glared into each other's eyes while their life blood drained from each of them. The same look, eyes full and bulging with rage, mirrored in each of their eyes. The furious glare melted into a last great gasp, spilling great globs of blood down from both men's mouths before both fell, their eyes still bearing the look of pure rage in death.

Spalding recognized the rage. He saw it many times in battle. The rage born of the demon of war. All men wore it, living and dead in battle. All warriors shared it. It locked men's eyes in a tunnel vision to their immediate front in battle. Men's brains seemed to pour from their ears in the height of battle. They only looked to their immediate front, for in that moment all of life and death faced them, demanding their full attention. Their blood flowed hot in their veins in such moments. They thought of nothing else. They left the larger sense of the battle to their captains. In their captains they trusted to deliver them from the madness and hell that is the fury of battle.

It all shone clear to Spalding in this instant. In this instant of madness and mayhem, of men screaming for the last time in this explosion of rage called war. Of men dying by one another's hand. All they are, were, and hoped to be yanked away in this moment of rage; of battle. The terrible responsibility of leading men in battle choked his breath away for a moment, but in an instant flittered away to clear thought. A plan immediately flowed through his mind. He suddenly felt alive and fully awake, staring down in wonder of his hands reloading his pistol without any conscious thought of his own. God's will, he thought, turning to Sweeney.

Sweeney stumbled backwards along with the rest of the line, swearing many an oath and waving his sword in the air. "Call your men to my support!" he yelled to Spalding.

"Wait!" Spalding said, "look about! Look to their rear! They are advancing with little regard for it! They are pushing us into this swale! If they keep moving the same way, I can take half my men through the woods to their left, and strike in their rear, along with Stoddert's men, envelop and surround them and cut them to pieces! What's left we'll drive into the river! I've got to get around their rear!"

Sweeney let his sword fall to his side, scanning the madness engulfing him. Divide in the face of a superior foe? What nonsense ran through this Wyoming officer's mind? He gazed at Spalding firing his pistol and waving the spent weapon to the ridge on their right. Through the wisps of smoke men poured to the top of it, starting to lay down their own fire into the enemy. Hartley's and Murray's men! Now Spalding's plan made all the sense in the world. "Yes! By God! Yes! We can turn their own momentum against them! I'll send a runner to Colonel Hartley!" Sweeney gasped.

"No time for that!" Spalding said, gazing at the mounted man darting about the men forming on the ridge. "If we're to act we need to act now!" he added. "I reckon the good colonel's already figured out what we're about anyhow! He's already starting to enfilade them! We've got to move!"

Sweeney stole a glance up to the ridge and back to the enraged line of Indians darting about to his front and firing at his line. One of his men twirled about and fell to his side, almost bringing him down with him. A ball whizzed by his ear. "You're right Captain!" he screamed at Spalding. "Get to it! We'll hold here, be damn quick about your movement!"

Spalding nodded. Firing once more he ran back to his men,

confident of his plan. This time the Indians advanced up the center. This time their confidence and impetuosity turned against them. Wyoming in reverse, Spalding thought, pouring down upon his veteran fighters and barking out commands. "Odds with me!" he shouted over the roar of rifles and muskets, referring to his earlier division of his men into ones with odd and even numbers. "Evens with Jenkins!" All obeyed immediately, recognizing the potential of the movement just as clearly as their captain. The taste of revenge wetted all their palates. They thirst for it ravenously, feeling this time it would be quenched.

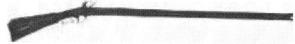

Chapter Fifty-Five

Elliot and Terry gained the tree line to the rear and right of their Division, carefully advancing into it. Both held their long rifles at the ready and darted from tree to tree, one covering the advance of the other. After advancing a rod or two Elliot stopped behind a tremendous tree, waving Terry to his side. "They've cleared out," he whispered to his partner, peeking his head around the tree, assessing their situation.

"They've got a wounded man slowing them, if we run like deer I think we can cut them off before they gain their friends' company again." he said, turning and looking sternly into Terry's eyes.

Terry looked back to the smoke drifting through the tree's behind them and listened to the sounds of the brisk fight to their rear, considering Spalding's orders.

"He said to clear it!" Elliot said. "They're Tory rats, turned against family and home! If we go back for help they'll escape. We've got a chance here man! I know you Terrys despise the Tories more than most, if'n that's possible," Elliot said, watching Terry consider his words.

Terry's cold eyes stared back at him. His reference to his brother Parshall stung him deeply. What of it? Was he responsible for his brother betraying their ranks and joining the enemy? He thought not, and damn anyone who did. Didn't Elliot hear the story of Parshall seeking him out on the day of the Battle of Wyoming? No doubt remained to his purpose upon finding him. The story of John Pensil slaying his brother Henry after finding him hidden on an island in the river rang true and deep to him. This war tore families and friends asunder. Its great purpose and meaning even rose above the sacred call of family. Its higher meaning changed the hearts of many, leaving lifelong friendships devastated in its wake. That purpose, either for or against, burned with equal intensity in the souls of the men on either side of it. A chance lay here to strike at the foe. He swore an oath to himself right then and there to fire no matter who's face shone down his rifle's sights. His sense of duty demanded it. "Lead on, damn it!" he said to Elliot. "Lead on!"

Both men dashed around the tree, running madly through the forest to gain ground. In a few rods Elliot stopped, pointing down to a slight clearing between the trees running almost down to the river. The telltale sounds of the battle quickly mapped out the position of their foe in his mind. "They'll have to cut across this clearing to get back to their lines!" he said, "let's hope we've not missed the rats."

Terry nodded, leaning back against the tree Elliot hid behind. Both checked their rifles then leveled them on the clearing. They waited, not moving a muscle, lest it betray their presence.

Now and then a spent ball spilled through the leaves around them, rolling and tumbling to the earth. Some smacked into trees, rolling down the bark to the ground. Both ignored the sounds, intently listening and searching the edge of the clearing for a rustle or movement in the brush to the left of the clearing. Just as the muscles in their arms started burning from holding up their long rifles so long a twig snapped.

An Indian, painted half red and half black from head to foot, carefully stepped into the clearing.

Both men stared down the sights of their rifles at the Indian brave looking about, but held their trigger fingers still, knowing more followed. They watched the whites of the Indian's eyes dart to and fro, ready to dispatch him if his eyes locked with theirs. Bigger bucks follow in the herd, wait them out.

The bigger the buck, the bigger the trophy. To their relief, the warrior turned and slightly waved the barrel of his rifle to his rear. Several white men in green coats and hunting shirts slowly stepped into the clearing. None looked about, trusting the keen eye of the Indian to their own. One, two, three, then finally four stepped out, all casting a nervous look behind them before scampering down the clearing to regain their line of battle.

Elliot cocked his eye from the barrel of his rifle over to Terry. "Wait until the last," he whispered ever so slightly, "we'll get the last, they're too great in number to chance getting them all. Let them clear out. The biggest buck is always the last of the herd!"

Terry stood firm, letting the silence of his firelock speak to his comrade's request. He searched every face of the white men, half hoping one of them shined familiar to him, while at the same time not wishing to know what face would catch his ball. But all bore the taint of treason, regardless.

Two more enemy rangers stumbled into the clearing, each with a wounded man's arm over their shoulders. A civilian stepped behind them, fanning his rifle around, not seeming to share the rangers' confidence in the Indian's eye. Another pair of rangers stepped out to their rear. All stopped to catch their panting breaths for a moment.

The civilian remained tense and on guard.

"Secord himself," Elliot whispered on a harsh breath. Both he and Terry watched the elder Secord's eye skirt the trees. To their dismay the Tory's eyes locked with theirs'.

Both watched Secord's jaw drop in disbelief. Before the stunned Tory could mutter a word or raise his rifle to his shoulder flames burst from the tree. A ball whizzed past his ear, slightly creasing it before thudding into the shoulder of the ranger behind him. The ranger's feet flew straight in the air, sending him groaning and rolling head over foot behind Secord. Another twirled about just to his side, clutching his arm.

An uncontrollable sense of panic raced through Secord's veins. Instantly raising his rifle, he fired blindly at the tree before turning and scattering into the trees opposite the clearing.

Elliot and Terry ignored the ball thudding into the center of the tree, calmly reloading their weapons. A few more balls whizzed past them from the firelocks of the few remaining Tories, but most of their number, including the Indian, scattered down the clearing or into the woods. The few remaining quickly tried reloading their weapons.

Terry stared resolutely at the panicked men, searching their faces, despite his oath. He recognized one, Moses Mount, another traitor from Wyoming, but the others remained clouded by distance and their rash movements.

"I'm ready," Elliot reported from the opposite side of the tree.

Terry looked down at his fingers instinctively going through the motions of loading his firelock while his mind and soul pondered his haunting thoughts. "Ready!" he answered Elliot's call, raising his rifle to his shoulder.

All of the Tories' eyes widened at the sound of the voices. One pulled his weapon up to his shoulder and pulled back the hammer, only to be cut down by Elliot's shot. He collapsed onto the ground to the horror of his friends. One grabbed him by the cape of his hunting shirt and his belt, roughly dragging him clear of the angry balls of the Rebel marksmen. The other wounded men hobbled along behind them, terrified and with a love of life fueling their hasty steps. Two Tories stood firm, raising their weapons to fire back at the Rebels to cover their wounded comrades' retreat.

Terry leveled his rifle on one of them and fired, sending him reeling about and tumbling to the ground.

Elliot huzzaed at the shot. "It's a turkey shoot for sure!" he screamed, quickly reloading his own piece. A ball splattered into the tree just by his head, sending splinters into his cheek. "No," he muttered, raising his rifle to his shoulder to fire at the last Tory dragging his wounded comrade down the clearing, vainly trying to gain distance before the Rebels reloaded. "It's a damn Tory turkey shoot!" His cheek stinging and his eye tainted with a slight trickle of blood, he aimed and fired nonetheless, his ball cutting a scrub oak in twain just to the side of the retreating Tory.

The Tory looked back, his wide-eyes betraying his absolute fear. Still, he tightened his grip on the cape of his wounded comrade's hunting shirt and dragged him along, cursing, but not abandoning the man.

"You ready or what?" Elliot asked Terry, wiping his eye free of the blood. He fumbled with a cartridge, cursing the trickle of blood flowing into his eye. "Fell the Tory bastard afore he escapes!" he screamed.

Terry took careful aim at the wide-eyed Tory, seeing in his eyes many a peaceful day hunting and fishing along the banks of the Susquehanna in his youth. Many a trap had been laid between the two. Many a wrestling match. Many a meal enjoyed by both of them prepared by the hands of their dear mother. They had grown and lived together, sharing all the cold winters by the hearth, and many a summer's day swimming in the creeks and rivers. They had courted the same women and stood beside each other at weddings. They had grown through life together. They were brothers.

Now it came to this. Brother against brother. Oh, what would their mother say if his hand pulled the trigger and released the ball that cut down her son, even if he did betray her? Wars do not last forever. How is one to mend the broken hearts left in its wake by such acts of pure vengeance? How is one to live with himself?

"Fire, damn it, afore he gets away!" Elliot screamed again from the other side of the tree. He raised his own weapon, fumbling to prime the pan through the blood trickling into his eye.

Terry clenched his finger against the trigger. All of the innocence of his youth flashed before his eyes in a great puff of white smoke exploding from the end of his rifle. Another blast sounded from the opposite side of the tree, adding to the smoke. He blinked, waiting for it to clear. Lowering his rifle, he peered into the clearing. The back of the wounded ranger disappeared into the brush by the side of the clearing. A hat still spun in the wild rye grass of the clearing behind him.

"You just missed the rat!" Elliot said. "But you took the hat right off his head! I could swear I saw him wet his britches!" He leaned against the tree, put another cartridge to his lips and bit off the top of it. "Best load," he said to Terry, noticing he stood deathly still by the tree side.

Terry nodded and slowly loaded his piece, all the while watching the clearing in awe.

"We wounded a few," Elliot said with pride. "They felt Wyoming lead for sure and I reckon they dare not come back for more!"

"Yes, they felt it fer sure," Terry said, proud of knowing he could perform his duty no matter what the circumstances. Finally, the answer to a question which plagued him ever since his brother's defection to the enemy rang true. He mused over the bridge in a man's soul from sense of duty to conscience, from soldier to civilian, and wished this war to end before another such test tortured his own soul again. He knew many shared his wish, but the war loomed far in front of them, overshadowing any thoughts of the future and that long ago time of peace. Too many scars and open wounds remained for it to ever truly heal, he thought.

"Best get back to the fighin' proper," Elliot said, ripping a length of cloth from his ragged hunting shirt. He handed it to Terry. "Bind my head?" he asked. "One of them just missed me, struck the tree and splinters got me."

Terry took the cloth, neatly tying it around his partner's head. The fury of the battle intensified to their rear, hastening his efforts to bind the wound. "Can you see to shoot?" he asked.

Elliot wiped the blood from his eye with his sleeve and smiled. "Damn right I can!" he answered. "And I intend to, this ain't over yet! Don't you hear that storm? It's the worst of all, the storm of war!"

"Yes," Terry said. "And I feel it a might bit in my soul."

A rustle to their rear brought both of the men's rifles up and ready for action. They lowered them in relief at the sight of a great elk cresting the hillside behind them. It strode a few steps forward and stopped, sensing the men. Snorting, it huffed away into the forest.

"There goes meat for a whole winter," Elliot said, shaking his head. Both of the men sighed in relief and prepared to trot back to their company when another beast appeared in the same place the elk vacated a moment ago. This beast bore a stern-faced soldier on its back. It trod painstakingly up the hillside, purely exhausted and played-out, but forced on by its determined master. The man on its back lowered his pistol, recognizing the two men. He turned on his mount, gesturing down the slope.

A dozen or so men ran up the hillside, barely pausing to nod at the Wyoming men. A half dozen Light Horse rode alongside of them. Both Elliot and Terry stared oddly at arrows sticking in some of the horses' flank muscles. They bobbed with each movement of the muscles, appearing as some grotesque ornaments of battle.

"You think they would have the decency to pluck those arrows out," Terry said under his breath at the fast moving group weaving through the trees.

"They would if it wouldn't cause them to bleed so," Elliot said. "If they yanked them now, while they're still at work, the blood would pour from them and bleed them out in no time. Have to do it when they're calm and out of this. It's the only way."

"Do you reckon we should join them?" Terry asked. "Looks like they're trying to gain the rear."

Another rush of movement to their left caught their eye before Elliot responded. They recognized the men moving among the trees immediately. "There's our lot," Elliot said, "we best get back to them, for it appears the tide of battle is turning and we're all going to strike to their left and rear!"

Both men trotted to rejoin their ranks, eager to strike again at their brazen enemy, confident this time victory lie with them. This fight they had to win, or certain death awaited them all, and each man seemed to sense it. Thus, both Elliot and Terry muttered a quick prayer under their breaths, beseeching God in all his mercy to deliver them from this macabre place and back to their homes some fifty odd miles below on the Susquehanna, and away from this nightmare. This living nightmare.

Chapter Fifty-Six

Captain-Lieutenant Sweeney counted the moments under his breath, hoping he had allowed enough time for Spalding to place his men on the flanks of the enemy and to his rear. The fire to their front increased, driving them back a rod or two in spite of Hartley and Murray men's covering fire from the ridge. Even Spalding's men lost a little ground, despite their bold efforts and staunch example of the brave lieutenant in their charge. Upon each rush of the enemy he led his men in a bold countercharge, driving them back, only to have them lunge back at them again in a few moments.

After a particularly hard rush Sweeney knew he had no more time. A quick, sharp, and simultaneous click turned his worried eyes about. He heard it before on the battlefield. It always brought chills down his spine. He stared at the sea of bayonets now glistening beneath the tapestry of nature's beauty on the ridge. The gold, red, and orange leaves flitting in the smoke-tinged breeze somehow added to the desperation of the action. His wary eyes followed the line of men on the ridge until they locked with eyes of equal determination. Knowing it to be too late to send a runner scampering up the hill by the increasing wails and whoops to his front; he found his answer in Colonel Hartley's cold eyes. Charge!

He raised his sword high, ready to order an all-out charge when new and somehow more distinct war whoops sounded to his left. Along with them a new burst of fire poured into the enemy's flank, sending them falling back in confusion. Sweeney peered through the clearing smoke at the line of men emerging as if from nowhere on his left.

He immediately recognized the three men hooting and yelling in front of the line. A smile grew across his face at Captains Boone and Brady, along with Lieutenant King. He looked up the ridge to Hartley, who apparently saw them too, for he waved his sword madly over his head yelling, "Drive them! Drive them! Drive them into the river!"

Sweeney screamed a great war whoop of his own and swung his sword forward. Drawing a deep breath, he stepped in front of the line yelling, "Charge! Charge! Charge the Copperheads!"

His war whoop echoed along the line like a contagion, joining the already screaming men of Hawkins, Brady, and King. Hartley's and Murray's men joined the whooping advance, spilling down the ridge and rushing steadily into the enemy's faltering line. Jenkins' men added their own cries down the line to Spalding and on to Stoddert with the Light Horse.

Wide and anxious Indian eyes peered all about, suddenly realizing their exposed position. "*OONAH*! *OONAH!*" rang down their ranks, their unmistakable call for retreat. They spilled from the swale like a liquid through a funnel into the gap in the rear between Captains Spalding's and Stoddert's men.

Hartley spurred his horse ahead, galloping through his victorious troops, swinging his sword wildly over his head, beseeching them to press forward with all due haste lest the enemy pour through the rear of the trap. The troops answered his call, running pell-mell into the retreating red men, slashing, clubbing, and shooting those unfortunate enough to be caught by the impetuosity of their charge.

To the rear Spalding yelled for his men to close up and join the men to their right, but to no avail. For the exhaustion and fatigue of their forced marches finally caught up with them, slowing them just enough to get but a few passing shots into the trees at the painted devils. The Light Horse, their mounts totally exhausted as well their riders, dashed in between the scattering red men in the trees, firing their pistols and swinging their sabers at the confused braves.

Stoddert, his men barely settled before the rush of retreating red men hit them, fired and fought a few luckless souls, but most slipped through his scattered ranks. Alas, they fared no better than the Wyoming Rangers, but gained a certain satisfaction upon witnessing the brazen and previously undefeated warriors of the Six Nations scurry away in defeat. The Rebel's victory could not be denied. They gained the field of battle. They drove the enemy.

The report of rifles and muskets soon faded along the mountainside above the mighty Susquehanna. On its high meadows men lie squirming in agony. Among its ancient trees brave warriors, both white and red, breathed their last.

Nonetheless, a wave of relief rushed over the exhausted victors of the battle.

A wave of disbelief ran through their vanquished foe.

After the last report of a firelock most of the victorious Rebels collapsed in exhaustion, both man and beast. They sat among the debris of battle, staring at the lifeless souls littering the field. Bloody and torn skull caps lay beside tri-cornered hats and wide brimmed slouch hats. Haversacks and pouches decorated with glittering pieces of silver and colorful porcupine quills speckled the ground. Broken firelocks sat side by side broken spears. Bent and broken swords littered the grass along with tomahawks. The unmistakable red color of blood peppered the leaves and matted the grass. All had been a hubbub just a moment before; now all sat still and quiet as death hovered over the field of battle searching for one more victim to claim among the groaning wounded.

Hartley slowly rode among the troops, too exhausted to issue any orders at the moment. They had done enough, he told himself, let them catch their breaths, they at least deserved that courtesy.

He, of course, felt disappointment that a lack of coordination allowed the enemy to escape, but they had barely done so, he reassured himself. Still, his mind played with the thought of driving them into the river. There they could have shot them like sitting ducks as the Tories and Indians had done to the men of Wyoming in the late battle. But no more could be asked of such men. They had trudged over impossible ground at the rate of twenty to thirty miles a day. Few could match that achievement and he knew it.

He sagged down in the saddle and watched Hooker Smith already tending to the wounded, directing men to carry this one or that one away, and to comfort others. He looked to the curious eyes of the preacher and his throng of women and children watching from the ridge, their eyes bearing a sense of wonder and disgust. Still no one, save Smith, spoke.

Captain Carberry rode his tired mount to Hartley's side and plopped down from the saddle, careful to avoid the arrows still sticking in the horse's flanks. "We did it," he reported. "They are on their way to Hell or Tioga, and they aren't looking back!" He collapsed to his knees, breathing deeply.

"Very well, Mr. Carberry," Hartley said. "You and your horsemen have behaved very admirably, as have you all. Every man performed well this day and I will be sure to mention you all most favorably in my report to Congress."

Boone, Brady, and King approached him, dipping their hats to him in salute.

"It is good to see you gentlemen have recovered from your lameness," he said with a slight smile. "Gentlemen, you and your men showed up at the precise moment you were needed and in the exact spot you were needed. Your vigor added to this victory, and I myself, am most grateful."

All three men nodded their heads to him.

"Now," Hartley continued, "if you would be so kind as to find a place in your canoes for the wounded, I would be most grateful." "Certainly, sir," Captain Brady said.

"Very well, see Doctor Smith, he shall direct you." He bowed his head slightly to the men doffing their hats to him, riding back to the men staggering into the field from the rear. He rode to Stoddert and doffed his own hat to the man before he could salute. "Mr. Stoddert, you, sir, deserve the esteem of your country!" He bowed his head to the man and also to Captain Spalding. "Captain Spalding your exertions shall be duly noted in my report to headquarters. You all acquitted yourselves with reputation. You all behaved well to a man! You have your country's gratitude! Most certainly!"

Spalding bowed his head to the colonel, rubbing his unshaven chin. "We best get moving, Colonel," he said. "We may have run off this lot but the whole Six Nations may be about Chemung now."

"Yes, quite," Hartley said. Looking around at the played-out men and horses and muttered, "Do you think they're up to it?" under his breath.

"They have to be," Spalding said. Stoddert bobbed his head in agreement.

"Very well, assemble the men and we shall be off, there are still some fifty miles between us and relative safety. There certainly is no safety here. We shall have to let the dead bury the dead, I'm afraid."

"Yes sir," both men said, doffing their hats in salute.

"By the way, Captain Spalding," Colonel Hartley said, pulling back on the reins of his mount to momentarily face the frontier officer, "does this place have a name?"

"Yes sir," Spalding quickly answered, gazing about the field of death. "We call it *Indian Hill** around these parts, sir."

"Yes, quite appropriately named to say the least," the colonel answered with a nod, reining his mount around one of the dead painted men. "Quite!"

The battle had been won, but the gauntlet still lay wide open between them and safety, and every man, woman, and child knew it from the preacher to young Lord Butler and George Palmer Ransom, drummer and teenage son of the late Captain Ransom killed in the Battle of Wyoming.

This day the young soldier struck a blow of revenge for his father. For certain one brave lay dead on the field, felled by his ball. But this day, this victory, would not be complete until they reached Wyoming, nor would his thirst for revenge be quenched until more fell by his hand.

Wyoming tasted a little revenge this day, but they yearned for more than a taste, much more.

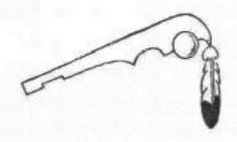

*Note: Indian Hill is located near present Laceyville, Pennsylvania

Chapter Fifty-Seven

"*Van der Lippe's* farm," a Wyoming scout reported to Colonel Hartley. The colonel leaned against the pommel of his saddle, staring at the abandoned farmstead spreading out in front of them in the pale moonlight. Though the cabin sat burned to ashes part of the barn roof remained held up by a few charred, but solid beams. A few of the outbuildings appeared serviceable also.

Hartley leaned back in his saddle, gazing at the weary souls trudging along the trail and to the moon shining brightly in the early evening sky above them. "We shall make camp here this night," he announced. "By my recollection we have come some thirteen or fourteen miles on this day's march. With two skirmishes and a pitched battle, I say we have come far enough." He threw one leg slowly over his saddle, gently sliding down to the ground. His aching feet burned. "Yes," he said, "we shall definitely camp here this night. One of you scouts signal the canoes to pitch here for the night. It shall give Smith time to treat the wounded. Tell him of our plans." "Yes sir," a scout said, rambling off to the river-bank.

"Captain Bush," Hartley said, turning his head to the officer sagging in the saddle behind him. The officer lifted his head up, pushing his hat from over his eyes. "See that a strong guard is posted."

The tired officer nodded his head and barked some orders to the ranks stumbling behind him. Two sergeants loudly repeated his order. Under the unforgiving eye of a staunch corporal several reluctant men marched from the ranks to the perimeter of the farm. The corporal promptly posted them, giving each a stern look warning them to remain vigilant.

The remaining column of men, women, children, pack-horses, livestock, and oxen, slowly spread out on the fields around Van der Lippe's farm. Women lifted sleeping children down from perches atop pack-horses. Other women carrying children in their arms slid down from the backs of moaning oxen.

The Light Horse gathered near the barn, immediately constructing a makeshift corral to tend to their wounded mounts. Arrows still protruded from several of their flanks. They neighed and whinnied while saddles and blankets slid from their sore backs.

Fires promptly lit the entire plain. Soon their flames danced in the night sky, sending great bursts of sparks high into it. Their crackle brought a sense of comfort and security to all.

Hartley walked up to one of the fires staring blankly into its flames, his mind full of thoughts of the day and the day to come ahead. Plopping down to sit, he barely noticed Colonel Denison walking up to him.

Denison eased his rifle down to the ground and took off his hat, wiping his sweaty brow with his arm. Exhausted, he plopped down next to the fire and joined Hartley. His eyes followed Hartley's to the flames.

"Wondrous, isn't it?" Hartley asked, rolling an eye to Denison. Such reflection on the mysteries of life eased his mind of the troubles of the day.

Denison said nothing. He too let his mind drift into the heavens with the flames. The face of a lad standing on the other side of the fire tore his eyes from the flames. He raised an eyebrow and asked "What is it Lord?"

"Sirs," Lord Butler said, easing his way around the fire. He held something loosely wrapped in a cloth. "I have your ration of beef." he added, passing the cloth to Denison.

Looking to the fire he scratched his head, finally deciding he hungered too much to attempt to reheat the boiled meat. Besides, taste mattered not on expeditions such as these; only nourishment. Hastily unwrapping the chunk of beef, he ripped off a piece, immediately gnawing on it. Tearing off another piece, he handed it to Hartley.

"I am sorry but the whiskey is spent," Lord said. "But no one has gotten sick from the water, yet, that is." He handed the men his canteen. "Filled it from the well," he explained. "It should be good. And by the way, all the flour is gone, too."

Neither of the men said a word. Their eyes blank and empty, they continued pondering the flames and gnawing on the tough meat.

Lord noticed their fascination and cleared his throat. "Mr. Priestly has a new theory on *'dephlogisticated air'*," he said, Mr. Priestly refutes the theory that combustion is accompanied by the release of phlogiston. His work on the mystery of airs is quite interesting. It is a wonder what such great minds as he, and his friend Doctor Franklin, are dwelling on these days."

Hartley looked up from his tough meat and slowly to Denison. "Colonel Butler makes sure his children are well read, does he not?" he asked.

"Quite," Denison said, shaking his head at the lad. "To us it is just flames, lad," he said. "Some are content to leave the mysteries of God to God. But others fear not to seek his light in them. I say let them search, my day is too filled with life to dwell on such matters."

Lord smiled and bowed his head, graciously departing the fire to attend to his duties.

"He does a fine job as Quartermaster," Hartley said. "I'll give him that. As to Mr. Priestly and the great Doctor Franklin I shall take him at his word." They both chuckled. The sounds and groans of wounded men and frightened horses neighing soon quelled their sense of humor. Both men tore and gnawed at the incredibly tough meat and stared into the flames again. "I must say I am quite anxious to finally meet Colonel Butler face to face," Hartley said, swallowing a huge chunk of meat. "The page relays a man's thoughts, but alas, man is more than his thoughts alone. I look forward to meeting one whom sired such a fine lad. I shall also be glad in many other ways to finally reach Camp Westmoreland."

"I shall also be most glad, and I must say relieved to finally end this trek through the wilderness," Denison said. "Most assuredly," he added, lifting Lord's canteen up to his nose and sniffing its contents. Shrugging his shoulders, he took a long drink from it.

"Tastes fine," he said, passing the canteen to Hartley.

"We drank worse than this in Canada," Hartley said, taking a long drink. An ear splitting yell and a series of curses startled him, spilling some of the water from the canteen. He jiggled the canteen and jerked it from his mouth, dropping it to the ground. He bent down, looking over his shoulder to the makeshift shelter Hooker Smith had constructed to perform his duty as surgeon.

Denison stopped eating and peered back at the convulsing man held down by three other stout men while Hooker Smith stood over him. Another man forced a thick piece of tough leather between the patient's teeth, pleading with him to bite down tight onto it. The man's terrified eyes glowed in the eerie light, alive and full of intense fear. His cries crept through the leather thong.

A glint of yellow lantern light sparkled from the bloody blade of a saw shaking in Hooker Smith's hands. The doctor cursed, yelling for someone to wipe the sweat from his brow. Cursing and grabbing firmly on the man's leg with one hand, he steadied the blade, finally performing the necessary task amid muffled cries. The pale yellow light reflected in his grim eyes. He narrowed them in the light, full of intent to perform his duty.

The leather suddenly slipped from the man's mouth, letting all of his anguish ride on his loud cries. All became silent from the spine-tingling wails.

Hooker Smith's curses paled in the man's cries.

Finally, a gruff soul forced the leather back into the man's mouth, relieving all in the camp.

"There is always the surgeon's butchery after battle," Hartley said, letting his hand fall limp with the meat. He lifted his knees up to his chest. Bowing his head in between them he let the meat fall from his hand. On a harsh breath he whispered a prayer.

Denison, suddenly losing his appetite as well, rolled over, facing away from the surgeon's table. He stared at the dancing flames before him, thinking of the slain souls they left behind on the battlefield today. Listening to the man's tortured cries and pleas, he could not help but wonder who were the luckier; the dead or the wounded?

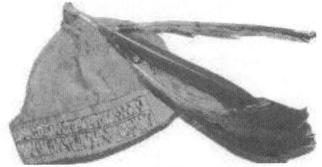

An actual Indian skull cap left on a battlefield along the Susquehanna River.

Chapter Fifty-Eight

Crowds of people gathered on the green at Wilkes-Barre, anxiously listening to the music of the approaching column. Colonel Butler ordered all of his men to form into two ranks on opposite sides of the road and waited patiently in between them, pacing back and forth and fidgeting with the hilt of his sword. His eyes remained locked on the road. His scouts reported the approach of the column two days ago and his imagination flashed with visions of their hardships. But they had won a major victory, burned four villages, and came back with tons of plunder and livestock. Quite an achievement to say the least, especially since every foot of the march lay in enemy territory for the most part. In fact, he had doubled the scouts and patrols in anticipation of the column's return. He would not fully breathe easy until they stood on the green before him. He looked to the cannon on the north end of the green, making certain the officer commanding it remained alert and ready for action.

The officer noticed his commander's stern gaze and barked a few expletives at his men. All stood taller after being dressing down by the officer. After he completed his tongue-lashing he looked to Butler, who nodded his head in confirmation of his actions. The sharp banging of drums and shrill of fifes turned his head back to the road. The haggard, but proud column, finally marched into view.

Hartley sat tall in saddle just ahead of the musicians. His eyes stared straight ahead and his stiff neck held his head high. Men in ragged and torn blue regimentals closely followed the musicians, led by the always regal and immaculate Captain Bush, though slightly tarnished. His regimental, cocked hat, and trousers stood out among the men, including Hartley, for showing little of the tears and soil so prevalent on the others' clothing.

Bright eyed civilians, liberated and glad of it, gazed upon their counterparts of the wilderness post with a strange fascination. The Wyoming civilians stared back for a moment, but most turned their eyes to the cattle, oxen, horses, and pack-horses loaded with plunder. Many clamored alongside of the plunder on the packhorses backs and cattle, trying in vain to recognize any of it as their own. The gruff actions of the Light Horse detailed to guard the plunder and herd the animals kept their fingers at a distance. A few harsh words announced their ire, but the sight of the proud Wyoming men marching with jutted chests and firelocks held tightly at their shoulders turned their critical words into a chorus of cheers. Captain Spalding graciously doffed his hat to the praise and thanks poured onto his men.

A voice from the river announced the arrival of a fleet of canoes, turning many eyes to it. A few anxious merchants, chief among them Mathias Hollenback, darted down to meet the canoes at the landing. He greeted and shook each of the men's hands departing the canoes, offering deep sympathy to the wounded souls lying prone in the canoe bottoms. Between his words of praise, he managed to drop in a few hints as to the value of the plunder. The answers he received brought a great smile to his face which quickly faded when one of the men told him with a fine smirk all could be obtained at auction, by the highest bidder. Hollenback burst into a rage, only quelled by the request of some of the men asking him to help lift the wounded from the canoes. After helping with a few of the moaning and suffering men, his tongue fell silent of complaints.

Mixed emotions followed the men of the expedition into camp. Many of the Wyoming people broke out kegs of whiskey, rum, and ale, of which each man gladly partook in consuming his fair share, but their haggard and careworn faces quelled any sense of celebration. They seemed just glad to be alive and free of the torturous marches and threat of Indians and Tories pouncing on them from any direction and at any moment. Most sank down onto their blankets around fires soon after setting up their camp, gladly accepting the many gifts of food offered to them from the grateful citizenry and the garrison.

Captain Bush even declined an invitation to dance, sighting his saddle sore backside as the main reason for his polite refusal. Disappointed women, newly arrived and hearing of the light-footed officer, graciously accepted his reason, with the stern promise of a dance the next night.

Hartley watched the crowd of disappointed women and chuckled, along with Nathan Denison. He noticed Colonel Butler turning his nose to it all. He eagerly shook the man's hand upon finally meeting him, but seemed a bit put-off with his no-nonsense manner. The man immediately asked for a full briefing of the whole expedition and seemed indifferent to the praise of his son, young Lord Butler.

In spite of it all Hartley accepted his invitation to use his quarters for the night and found the man most gracious when not under the eyes of his men. They dined, drank, and talked of small things, easing Hartley's mind of its troubles.

As Butler threw the last log on the fire in the hearth of his cabin and graciously offered a last toast, his eyes drew tight with the same dour look of earlier in the day. "For all your accomplishments, which are in themselves great and deserve much praise, I fear you have only given the Six Nations a strong slap when a full beating is called for. A slap may sting for a bit, but does little to hurt the foe, it only fuels their resolve, if anything." Sitting his mug down on the table he bowed his head to the exhausted colonel before walking over to the door. Lifting the latch, he stopped. Looking back over his shoulder he said, "I fear if Congress does not act by sending more reinforcements quickly they may find their frontier borders much lower than they expect." With that, he locked eyes with Hartley before slowly lifting the latch and excusing himself for the night.

A man of deep insight, Hartley thought, plopping down on a featherbed, and of true words. Despite the comfort of the bed after sleeping on the rough ground with barely a blanket to cover him from the rain and cold, Butler's words echoed through his mind. Yes, he thought to himself, if the enemy should take Wyoming, New York, Pennsylvania, and New Jersey will realize its importance too late. He reconsidered his own his plans he decided upon after the battle. Butler was right. It was not enough. He hoped Washington to be true to his word, and be quick to dispatch a larger expedition to this region. No, he would not depart for Philadelphia as he had planned. Too much danger still lay in these mountains, hills, and vales.

He would stay until it passed. Conscience demanded it of any man of honor. But at the same time his tired body made him realize mortal man only had so much to give. And he was indeed mortal, his aching body attested to that fact.

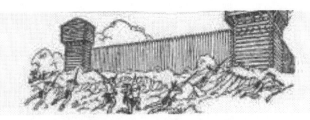

Chapter Fifty-Nine

The men settled into a state of calm for the last two days. Backs and feet welcomed the brief respite. Among the women hints of faint smiles gradually began to replace the dour looks of fear so prevalent on their faces as of late. Children, overjoyed by the new sense of calm, started playing again. Their chuckles and laughter once again resounded around Wilkes-Barre. Eyes looked away from war and to the domestic pleasures of life. The harvest occupied many conversations. Optimistic hints of planting for the next season ran among certain circles.

A faint ray of hope began to shine, and all welcomed it, though every heart still stopped beating upon hearing any suspicious sound and every eye darted to any sudden movement in the brush. All reassured themselves and each other against their apprehension, though. Colonel Butler's scouts would be sure to alert the settlement upon the first sign of trouble. Surely the enemy would not be so bold as to strike against these men in arms, now rested and well fed, men whom had given them such a thrashing in their own country. No, perhaps they had won at least a brief respite from the raids and constant harassment.

New praise grew for Hartley's little army on this almost full second day of peace. He accepted it in the spirit of hope shared by all, but deep down inside his soul he still cast a wary eye to the surrounding mountains, as did all.

But on this bright morning all seemed well, enough so he gracefully accepted Colonel Butler's invitation to stroll along the green. The two men slowly walked along the river, mindful of the pistols in their belts. Nonetheless, Hartley attempted to lighten the mood by sharing pleasantries and small talk.

But Butler seemed anxious, not of the lurking threat of the enemy, but rather of a something altogether different. As other minds thought of the harvest, planting and such, his mind fluttered with a grandiose dream as of late. Reaching a fine and clear spread of green grass he marched boldly about, taking wide steps as if surveying the land. Hartley grudgingly tried to keep pace with the man's spirited walk but finally stopped, letting Butler take a few more great strides before saying, "Yes, it would be a fine place for a new fort."

Butler's eyes lit up at the words. He turned, stretching his arms in a wide arc. "I am so glad you, a man of vision, see what I see," he said, taking a few more steps to one side and spreading his arms wide again. "Here shall stand the walls, solid, two rows of fine logs laying horizontally with a space between, six to eight feet, filled with well tamped down earth!" His eyes rose up the imaginary walls as if they already stood. Knowing his determination by the glitter in the man's eyes, Hartley had no doubt this vision would become a reality. He walked up next to him, nodding his head.

"Yes," Butler said, "thus formed the walls shall be carried to a full height of seven or eight feet! And all around the enclosure formed by the wall, a platform, or bench, will stand, enabling our men to deliver their fire over top the walls. All around the outside shall be a ditch, beyond that, an abattis, formed by setting firm the tops of pitch-pine trees, trimmed and sharpened by the axe, pointing outwards." He took a few more steps, waving his arms in a circle. "Here, an embrasure, along with several all around the walls, from which cannon may be fired! All the corners of the fort shall be rounded, as to give a sweeping arc of fire, and flank all sides! Inside the enclosure, which should be about a half-acre, barracks for the garrison."

He stopped once more and strode to the southeast, leaving Hartley standing and watching wide-eyed at his enthusiastic vision of the new fort. "Here shall run a timbered, and thus protected, access to a copious spring of water at the margin of the river, just as Forty Fort had." He took a deep breath, gazing up the river. "Two small blockhouses shall be constructed on the upper side of the fort, across the plain, to shelter those who cannot be accommodated in the fort proper." He took a step back toward Hartley and stared with sparkling eyes at the whole sweeping vision as if it already existed. "This shall be done before this month is finished. I know these men, my men, they all have strong backs and are up to any challenge. That they are! Besides, they know it may be paramount to our very survival, what with the lackluster response of Congress."

"Oh," Hartley said, "I assure you our greatest minds are considering the Wyoming question at this very moment. Such a great movement as they have planned shall take time. My little slap, as you call it, shall be nothing compared to the sledgehammer blow coming, I do most earnestly assure you, fine sir."

Butler looked at him with a raised eyebrow. He only hoped they survived to see the day of which the good colonel spoke. Both of the men stared at one another, gauging the sincerity of each other's words.

The report of several rifles abruptly broke their stare. Both men shuddered, looking anxiously across the river. War whoops echoed over the water. Screams of terror followed the whoops from the far bank, soon joined by women's cries of concern from the camp.

"My God, my God, they're back!" Hartley gasped. "Who did you send over there?"

"No one," Butler said. "Whoever they are, they are not of this garrison."

Hartley blanched. He had been too lenient for the past two days, letting his men roam and mingle with whoever and wherever. Now some poor unfortunates paid the price.

"I have standing orders none are to go to the west side of the river," Butler said, starting to turn back to the camp.

Hartley turned with him, meeting officers and troops rushing to meet them. "What is going on across the river?" he asked before any of them could speak.

"Four of Captain Murray's men crossed the river!" Captain Stoddert reported.

"Crossed the river?" Butler asked. "What in heaven's name for?"

"Wild potatoes, sir," Stoddert answered.

Hartley rolled his eyes, remembering the others killed outside Fort Muncy on the same quest. These damn Dutchmen and their lust for wild potatoes, he thought. Will they ever learn? "Follow me at the long trot!" he ordered, running up the riverbank. All of the troops and officers filed behind him. Upon reaching the crest of the bank they spread into a strong defensive line, all scanning the opposite bank for any sign of the men.

"You left a guard at the camp?" Butler asked Captain Spalding, who searched the opposite riverbank intensely with a spyglass.

"Of course, sir," Spalding said, keeping his eye to the glass. His hand immediately pointed to the opposite bank. "There!" he said, waving to the troops nearest him. "Stand ready!"

Both Hartley and Butler stared in the direction he pointed, along with all of the eyes of the troops.

A bush rustled on the opposite bank. Dozens of rifles and muskets leveled on the movement.

"Hold your fire!" Hartley ordered. "We know not if they be friend or foe! Just stand fast!"

A man burst from the bushes, spilling down the bank in a tussle of flailing arms and legs. Bareheaded and seemingly unarmed, he quickly stumbled to his feet. His wide eyes cast a horrified gaze over his shoulder before he plunged terrified into the swirling waters of the Susquehanna.

"Get to the canoes!" Butler ordered some men near him. "Get out to him before he's swept downstream!"

Several men darted down the bank to the canoe landing. Pouring into the canoes, they paddled madly into the river, rushing to the terrified and exhausted man swimming for his dear life.

The man plunged one arm after another into the water, his feet kicking up a storm of whitewater in his wake. He kept swimming headlong towards the opposite shore, either too terrified to stop, or not hearing the pleas of his rescuers to stop so they could pull him into one of the canoes.

He swam past the first canoe to the amazement of the officer within it. The officer bent down, barely missing the man's shoulder, his fingers running across a fresh red spot on the crown of the man's skull, trailing trickles of red in the water. Absolute terror shone in the man's bulging eyes.

The officer leaned back in the upsetting canoe, leveling it again to the relief of the men manning the paddles. He stared in horror at his fingers. What hell is at play here? he mumbled to himself. War cries raised his eyes to the approaching riverbank. "Drop those paddles and grab your muskets!" he ordered, calling to the next canoe to pluck the man from the water. He turned his eyes towards the scrub brush on the far bank. The stark and absolute terror in the man's eye flooded his mind's eye. Whatever caused it lay in wait there, waiting to pounce and strike. Their number could be legion or a half dozen. Whatever their number, these coldhearted killers waited just ahead of him and his men in their rickety birch bark canoes. They would not get them without a fight, though, he promised himself, drawing a pistol from his belt.

A call from behind broke his gaze at the riverbank. He looked back to the other canoes. Men waved them back and pointed to the far shore, shouting they had the man. Louder yells from the men watching from the far bank distinctly ordered him back across the river.

The men immediately replied to the order without word from their anxious officer, dropping their muskets and regaining their paddles.

Nonetheless, the officer nodded at the paddles splashing into the water, leveling his pistol at the bank until the canoe turned about in the swirling waters. His heartbeat stopped for the blinking of an eye from a glimpse of red paint and feathers through the brush. He lifted his pistol, intent on firing if he caught sight of the hellish demon again, even though he knew the devil to be well out of the range of his weapon.

"What?" the man grasping the rear paddle asked, increasing the rapidity of his movements upon noticing the glint in the officer's eye.

"Nothing," the officer muttered. "Just keep paddling!"

Chapter Sixty

"Poor man," Hartley said, watching the trembling man's lips trying to mouth an explanation of what he had experienced across the river. Butler stood staunchly beside him, quietly listening to the man mutter in German. Captain Murray bent over the muttering man, trying to take in all his words while Hooker Smith tended to the wound atop his head.

"Well, I don't know Dutch," Smith said, rising from the bed, "but it'll be best to let his wound air. He's been creased by a ball along his arm, as well. Hit on the head, too. He'll have plenty to tell his grandchildren after this is all said and done, though. He'll make it just fine, he will at that, but he'll be bald!"

The man ceased muttering, turning a grateful eye to Smith. He swallowed hard but managed to mouth a thank you before collapsing into the bed from pure exhaustion.

"Just doing my job, is all," Smith said with a smug smile. He collected his things and passed the two high ranking officers. "He'll be bald, in the most unnatural way, as I've said, but he'll live, there's worse things that could have befallen him." With that he excused himself, marching to the other beds in his makeshift hospital.

Murray slowly rose from the bed also, reassuring the man in his native tongue. The man's eyes opened wide. Tears streamed from them and he muttered, "Mien Goot! Mien Goot! Wildens!" after the officer. Another of Murray's men promptly took his place, reassuring the distraught man.

"Says they came out of nowhere, a full dozen of the rats, and struck them down before they could blink an eye," Murray reported to the officers. Both nodded. Hartley nervously rubbed his chin. Butler fanned his hand for the captain to continue. "He was keeping guard a few paces away from the others while they dug up the potatoes. The ball for him only creased his arm and he spun about. The savages in their bloodlust fell upon his luckless fellows, stabbing and firing point blank into their bodies, screaming like demons all the while. He rose, fired, and hit a large one in the shoulder. The big Indian barely moved in spite of the force of the shot. The other Indians swarmed down on him but the big one called them off, must've been some chief or somebody of importance, for they obeyed him. As they parted he marched through them with his war club raised and struck him down. He held up his rifle to shield the first blow, but the chief was so angry the blow splintered both the club and rifle. He stood with the two pieces of his splintered musket in his shaking hands when the chief struck him down with another club quickly passed to him. All he saw was stars and then he felt the cold earth beneath him. He felt the Indian's knee on the small of his back and a shearing sensation to his head. He said he heard a terrible ripping sound all along with the sensation, and realized it was the sound of his own scalp being torn from his head. The chief took a few steps back and held his bloody hair up, yelling and hooting for all get out when he saw his chance and bolted. The next thing he remembers is being pulled from the water. A hell of an ordeal to say the least."

"Indeed," Hartley and Butler both said at the same time.

"Thank you Captain," Hartley said. "You may return to your men. Tell your men, and all the volunteers from Northumberland, along with Captain Bush's company, to cook three days' provisions for the march to Fort Augusta." He pulled his watch chain and looked at the time piece in his palm, ignoring Colonel Butler's stunned gaze. "Be ready to march at four o'clock this day."

"Yes sir," Murray said, doffing his hat. He promptly turned and trotted towards his men, barking orders for all to hear. Surprised eyes all shot to the hospital before the booming voice of a sergeant scolded them to get about their duties.

Hartley put the watch back into his pocket, raising his lower lip. He rolled an eye to Butler. "I shall leave half my regiment here with you, sir," he said. He slowly stepped from the hospital, gazing sullenly at the mountains. Butler followed. "I am responsible for all the posts from Nescopeck to Muncy, and from thence to the head of the Penn's Valley. All of this vast frontier, from Wyoming to the far Allegheny Mountains. I have my little regiment, your men, along with two classes of Lancaster and Bucks County militia, barely enough, to say the least. If the Indians are bold enough to attack here, where the most men are assembled, what of the other posts spread all along the Susquehanna? I must attend to my duties sir."

Butler bowed his head, suddenly ashamed of his selfish nature. "Of course, Colonel," he said. "I understand."

"I shall return as soon as possible, Zebulon, most likely from Fort Jenkins, with provisions, cannon, and ammunition, if all goes well." He rubbed his eyes, sighing. "It is the best I can do, we must make do with the tools available. If there is an attack at Muncy or below, do not be surprised to receive orders to come to our assistance. But if not we must secure our posts for the winter. It is too late for another expedition even if we had fresh troops."

"Of course, the snow lays two feet thick when it comes and stays well into March," Butler said. "And we shall come immediately if called, if even by snowshoe, I assure you. All are grateful for your leadership on that incredible trek through the wilderness and tremendous victory at Indian Hill. It has done far more good than you realize. Perhaps more in men's souls than any other thing, but alas, that may be the most important thing, for in the end, all comes from the soul."

"Thank you, Zebulon."

"Of course, I would have liked to have accompanied you, but orders kept me at this post."

"We must all obey our orders, and I appreciate your understanding, for these troubles are not over, but may be just beginning anew."

"We shall raise the new fort before the month passes, I assure you. But it may be short of proper cannon. I shall await you to solve that problem."

"And I assure you all, I shall do my damn best."

"I know you shall."

"You men of Wyoming possess much grit and raw determination. As great as any I've ever encountered and the most determined belief in our country's cause. Even General Washington has commented upon it. I've heard him with my own ears. He is as proud of the Wyoming Rangers as I am. Be strong, as you always have against the foul winds blowing from every corner of the wilderness, for I promise you others do know of your struggles. Wyoming shall not fall as long as one of you breathes, I believe that with a heart as equal in patriotic fever as yours. Stand strong ye men of Wyoming! Stand strong and ye will live forever in the hearts of all men!"

Chapter Sixty-One

Chemung resounded with wails of triumph upon hearing a huge chief's boasts of slaying three Rebels and scalping a fourth. He paraded around the war post, thumping it with his war club with each new twist to his tale. Warriors whooped in delight when he raised several small hoops with hair stretched across them. Jutting his chest proudly, he pointed to a bruise and cut across his upper arm. A Bostonian's ball had grazed him but he did not even flinch when the ball struck, he bragged, adding how he fell upon the shaky white devil and fell him, lifting his scalp before his prayers to his demon God gave him the strength to run. He did not pursue him, though. He had his hair. He would claim the rest of the devil in due time. Now that he and the Seneca had arrived the shame of Indian Hill would be forgotten.

Gucingeratchton, brave war chief of the Seneca, strutted through the gathering of wide-eyed braves after his declarations and to his cabin, full of himself and his brave deeds of this day. Before entering the door held open by his beautiful wife, he turned, promising another strike at the white devils soon. The honor of the Six Nations demanded it. This time none of the lying Yankees would survive. The Yankees broke their solemn word and struck at the belly of the Six Nations like the cowards they are! Word of the white chief Denison joining the march infuriated him, he proclaimed loudly, especially since the white chief had promised not to raise arms against the Six Nations ever again. He lied! And this letter written by the white chief Hartley accusing them of killing and torturing women and children at Wyoming must be addressed! As all lies must! With that he turned, disappearing into the cabin with more hoots and whoops following him.

All did not share his enthusiasm, though, among them crestfallen Queen Ester herself. She watched the whole spectacle with a wary eye, a fear rising in her heart. A fear that all changed forever. A fear of the might she herself had seen in the cities of the white-eyes. Their numbers seemed endless. Their resolve made her wince. She braved a smile to the few curious eyes glancing at her before excusing herself. Turning, she strode slowly to the river. Its flowing waters always calmed her at such moments. She needed them now more than ever, she thought to herself.

Finding a grassy spot by the swirling Susquehanna she sat and watched it flow before her, wondering of the waters and of their great quest for the sea. She wished she could fling all her sorrows and concerns onto the waters and let them carry them far away. The world seemed to shrink around her and her people. No more could they freely canoe all the way down the river to the sea. No longer did the river seem a friend, but an enemy, carrying the settlements of the white-eyes along its banks. Oh, for the days of her youth when the vast expanse of land seemed too endless for any one people to claim for their own. The world had indeed shrunk: her world at least.

A nagging feeling at the nape of her neck broke her melancholy train of thoughts. She glanced out of the corner of her eye to a woman standing patiently behind her. She did not have to turn to see her whole face to recognize her.   "*Auweni*? Oh, Lydia," she said, bowing her head to face the waters again. She fought to hold back the tears threatening to spill down her cheeks. Raising her hand, she tried to slow the white woman's advance, ashamed of her tears. "*Alakqui*! You jogo," she said, "to Fort Niagara!"

Lydia stopped in her tracks, bowing her head.

"No safe for you and childs," Ester continued. "Much hatred, too much. *Quilawelelendam*!"

"Yes, I know," Lydia said, wanting to plead for her return down the river to Wyoming but knowing the fruitlessness of such a request. No one would be going down the river from Chemung but on a war footing. She looked to the river and to the great trees drooping their branches over it, sighing at the beauty of it all. She wondered just how that beauty compared to the cities marring the coastline, but quickly quelled the thought. You have been too long among the savages, she scolded herself under her breath, get a hold of your thoughts!

"You have been too long here," Ester said, hearing her faint whisper. "I done all I can for you. Young Secord, Cyrus, going Niagara, get more provisions, you jogo with him. *Vivre vieux!*"

Lydia's eyes widened upon hearing the good English rolling off the Queen's tongue, despite the intermingling French. In grief all things flowed more easily, she reasoned. "Yes," she said, wanting to reach out and take the Queen's hand to thank her but thinking better of it. This Indian Queen had destroyed their home and sent her men folk to who knows what hell in Canada. Now she sent her and her innocent children to the same fate. But at the same time she knew without the Queen's protection they would all have been killed or she at least separated from her children. That meant something. "Thank you!" she said on a gasp of emotion before turning away holding her hand to her cheeks to check her tears. She stopped a few steps away and turned, wishing to find better words to express her gratitude but none could pass the growing lump in her throat.

Ester heard Lydia stop and looked down to her own hands. They suddenly felt tainted with the grime and blood of vengeance. "They cry for vengeance! I have had vengeance with these very hands! Still it does little to ease the grief of my son's loss! Much blood has flowed, but none cleanses my heart of its pain! No! It will never! Jogo, dear Lydia, *par Dieu*! I hope you find Boss and be happy! Is all I can do! Jogo!"

Lydia took a few steps forward, reaching her hand down to the Queen. In the shadows on the Queen's face Lydia noticed glittering tears streaming down her cheeks before she gruffly rubbed them away with her arm. The bells and trinkets on her clothing jingled in a strange rhythm that seemed out of place.

"Jogo!" Ester demanded, waving her jingling arms behind her. "*Le mieux est l,ennemi du bien.*"

"I can hear the pain of your broken heart," Lydia said on a

whisper. "It flows to the waters and spreads across the very heart of the land. It weeps with your beleaguered soul. Once more I thank you, for I know you have done all in your power you could do. You are caught up in this as we all are; may God have mercy on all our souls!"

A cry of pure anguish poured from Ester's soul. She waved her arms behind her, fighting her tears to no avail. She collapsed face first into the grass, clutching it as a dear child just about to die. This land, as she knew it, as her people had known it for thousands of years, would change soon, and with that part of it would die, never to reborn but in the vague memory of its conquerors. She, nor no one, white or red, seemed able to stop it. Fear flooded her whole body. "*C'est dommage,*" she cried. "*C'est fait* ! *Frapp'e de stupor! Hartley foius-moi le camp*!" She wept profusely for the earth and her people. One way of life had to die to make way for a new one; one she feared more than death itself. This brought a grief that pulsated through her very being as if conjoined with the trembling earth itself.

She feared nothing but death itself could ease this grief. Nothing.

This revolution, as they called it, changed all. This revolution touched all, even the very earth itself. Nothing would ever be the same in its passing. Nothing, the whole world wide.

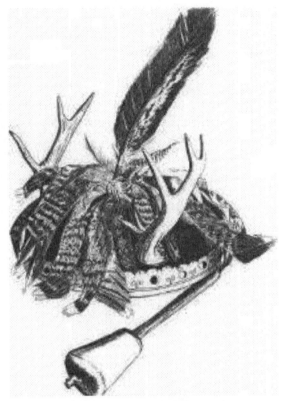

Chapter Sixty-Two

William Jameson looked about the land, taking in the full beauty surrounding him. Birds chirped, sitting on branches among the bright colors of Autumn's leaves. A few clouds drifted lazily through the blue sky. Breezes teased the ripe grain in the fields below him. All seemed at peace. Perhaps, finally, the Indians had holed up for the winter, he hoped. Anyways, he put off checking the conditions of things at the ruined homes of his brother and father in Hanover too long. Snow would fly soon, he felt its warning in the bite of the breeze cutting his cheeks. This had to be done, and now.

He heard the echo of axes and the crack of timber falling to his rear. He marveled on how the fort Colonel Butler had ordered built came along so famously. Almost all of the walls had been raised. By the end of the month it looked to be finished; meeting the colonel's goal he barked to the ranks each night after another hard day's toil. Their lives and future depended upon it, he told everyone so much they tired of hearing it. The Six Nations would not sit idle, he preached, come spring they would strike. How strong we stood against them depended entirely on how strong of a fort we had! Something in his words struck home, for everyone, including him, worked their fingers to the bone constructing the new Fort Wyoming.

The colonel's warning grew in credence in Jameson's mind upon sight of the burned and charred remains of homes he passed along the roadside. It sent chills down his back. Desolation amongst beauty, he thought, glancing down to the rifle laid across the saddle of his horse. His mount seemed to share his feelings, lifting its head and perking its ears, neighing loudly. He gently patted its neck, leaning forward to whisper reassurances in its ear. It calmed the beast, but only added to the tingle haunting the nape of his neck.

The truth of Colonel Butler's words again rang loudly in his mind. Looking behind him he thought of his friend Asa whom accompanied him for a while but turned back to the fort on some trifling excuse. Perhaps he should have gone with him, he mused for a moment, thinking of the Indians and Tories. They would be back. They had been back. Suddenly he felt totally alone and isolated. He eased back and looked over his shoulder, letting the sounds of those raising the fort reassure him.

Only a mile or so, he thought to himself, and you will be there. He carefully and slowly looked all around. Nothing moved in the trees or in the bushes. All seemed quiet, too quiet. No birds chirped. Only the caw of a spooked crow echoed among the dull thuds of distant axes. His eyes followed the black bird flying over his head. He wished for a moment to have its eyes and therefore its view, but quickly scolded himself for being so apprehensive. Colonel Butler ordered scouts to constantly patrol the whole valley and beyond; in fact, he reasoned, looking down at the fresh footprints in the muddy road, scouts preceded him no more than an hour ago. Too much real fear haunted Wyoming; do not add to it with an imaginary one, he thought.

He tightened the reins and gripped his rifle more firmly, nonetheless. Flicking his knees together against his mount's flanks; he increased its gait.

An overwhelming feeling stopped him at the crest of a slight hill. Before him the road meandered through a clearing before bushes funneled it to a crossing through *Buttonwood Creek*. The sugar bush seemed very thick along the funneling path to the crossing, he noticed for the first time. It apparently had never bothered he nor anyone else before; but now times had changed; everyone's eyes seemed a bit keener to such dangers. A savage could burst from the brush, do his terrible work, and disappear in the blinking of an eye. He must report these funneling bushes when he got back to the fort. This brush must be cut back because of the potential threat it harbored.

He scanned the brush ever so carefully, looking for the slightest movement. Reaching down, he cocked the hammer back on his rifle, ready to lift it and fire in an instant. His muscles tightened. He perked up in the saddle and looked all around, watching his horse's alert ears for any sign of distress or warning.

An enormous crack from a great falling tree rang through the air. His horse danced around to face the sound, almost felling him from the saddle. Scolding the beast, he tightened the reins in his fingers, balancing his wobbly rifle on the saddle again.

He reined his mount back towards the creek and looked around yet again; this time not for any savages, but for any friendly eye watching him. He would not want word of his overreaction and fumbling mount to get back to the fort. What would they think? With that he gritted his teeth and spurred his reluctant mount forward, despite its neighs of warning. "Be quiet," he said, spurring it to a trot by the bushes. "In a few more trots we'll be beyond it! We mustn't let fear of every bush cripple us!"

The words barely escaped his lips before a force knocked him from the saddle. He rolled head over heels into the mud, madly groping for his rifle through the stars flooding his vision. He stumbled to one knee, blinded by the mud in his eyes. Another whack struck his skull. He collapsed backwards, looking vainly through the mud at his retreating horse. Another strike knocked him full on his back. His head ached and burned. Mud oozed into his gaping wounds. Raising one of his wrists, he wiped the muck and blood from his eyes, only to see a painted demon bending down over him.

Bared teeth flashed across the hideously painted face. The glint of a knife blade sparkled in his eyes before he felt a sharp blade about his head. Instinctively, he burst to his feet, running. He clamored through the woods, ignoring the snapping branches in his face. His feet fumbled along rocks and fallen timber but never slowed in their quest for life. Screams and yelps sounded in his rear. A whizzing sound brushed by his ear, followed by the crisp report of a half dozen rifles. He ran for dear life, his mother, family, and all he held sacred.

Blinded by blood, ooze, and muck in his eyes, he focused on the thud of the axes and ran towards the noises. For life waited among them; along with safety and freedom. He ignored the pain, but suddenly plowed into the trunk of a tree. He wheeled around it and kept plodding forward; he had too! The yelps grew fainter in his rear. The axes sounded more crisp to his front. Soon the groan of oxen and the familiar rhythm of men's voices grew along with the thuds.

He stumbled forward, now alert to the many pains about his body. His shoulder burned and felt wet with blood. His fingers crept up his shirt to find a hole in his flesh, but it did not compare to the sheer and agonizing pain about his head. He felt air on parts of his body he knew should never feel such sensations while he lived. It felt strange among the pain; a sensation he knew few ever felt. It scared him down to his toes. Tears cleared his eyes. His mouth mumbled "Mother, Mother," through his fluttering lips. The sounds of safety grew closer.

He ran and ran, collapsing when the sounds of safety boomed in his ears.

Gasps and shouts of alarm flooded his ears. The sound of rushing feet closed around him. Shock and disbelief hung on every word of his familiar language but he did not care. Safety lay with their tones, along with the hope of dear life.

"What is that he is mumbling," one voice asked close to his ear.

"Is it Mother?"

"What's about his skull? His brain?" another shocked voice asked.

"Back! Back!" another strong voice boomed. "Clear the way!"

Through his pain he recognized the voice of Hooker Smith and never thought he would be so glad to hear the boisterous doctor's voice again. "Save me," he begged through his delirium. "Save me." "What's that?" a voice asked. "What's that he's saying?" "He can speak?" another voice asked in astonishment.

"Yes!" Hooker Smith's voice boomed. "Now shut up so I can hear what he's asking!"

All fell silent. He felt a hand gently lift his head by the back of his neck and heard a sudden gasp.

"What is it son?" the voice belonging to the hand asked. He felt the hairs from the man's head bending down to hear his faint words on his lips.

"Save me, dear doctor, save me," he muttered on a tortured breath. Feeling the hairs lift from his lips, he opened his eyes to see the shocked doctor's eyes mirroring horror.

The doctor shook his head and gently nodded, noticing his gaze mirrored in the man's terrified eyes. "Of course, son," he muttered. "Of course."

The doctor carefully lifted him to an awaiting cart. "Be gentle as you can!" he called to the driver. "And you," he ordered the man cradling the shattered skull. "Be mindful of his head, that's his very brain oozing out from that tomahawk wound, keep it still, and bandaged, for God's sake!" The man nodded and the cart slowly pulled away.

Hooker Smith stood trying to catch his breath for a moment. Many surrounding him did the same. He reflected on the sheer horror of Jameson's ordeal and wondered of the man's great strength. "My God," he finally said, "if he can be saved, I will save him, for if a man wishes to live so badly, well, he shall." He climbed onto the saddle of his awaiting horse, silently knowing the brave man's wounds to be mortal. But one must keep faith, he reasoned, looking to the sea of shocked faces around him. The isolation of their settlement in the middle of this harsh wilderness loomed in each man's soul.

"We must keep faith," he said, turning his mount to follow the cart. "For faith is all Wyoming has, now. All we have is faith and one another."

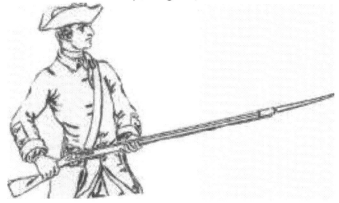

Chapter Sixty-Three

Colonel Hartley stood on the platform surrounding Fort Muncy's walls calmly surveying the land. The sun rose slowly over the trees from the east, its bright rays already threatening the frosty air and grass. Bright leaves danced on the breeze in the tall trees. The river shone brown with wisps of crisp fog about its face. Bald Eagle Mountain stood regally in the distance, its splendid grandeur overshadowing the landscape. Smoke rose from the chimney of the stone fort of Wallis, beckoning him with its promise of warmth and good food. But he stood firm, being a good example to the men bustling about in the early morning.

A loud crash turned his head to look below the platform. A huge hewn log tumbled to the ground with the curses of Captain Walker's men following it. Walker himself walked over and put his foot atop the log, reassuring his men and ordering them to lift the log into place again. "Winter's a coming," he said on a frosty breath. "The sooner we get these barracks done the quicker we'll be out of those damn ragged tents about Wallis' and around our own warm hearths. Now let's get to it!"

Hartley watched the men eagerly return to their work. The log quickly rose into place to the cadence of their work song. The call for more echoed through the gate to the oxen team pulling another log through the open gate.

These men had heart, if nothing else, Hartley observed, watching them work enthusiastically in their threadbare uniforms and small clothes. He shook his head and reminded himself of the pleas he had sent to Congress for provisions, pay, and clothing. Only ammunition came in abundance so far, but he had received promises. Promises do not fill bellies and clothe backs, though, he thought. No, they do not, fine gentlemen of Congress.

The sharp rap of a drum tore his eyes to two squads of men parading at the far end of the stockade. He looked with pride at the two officers drilling the men; sergeants recently promoted to ensigns for their distinguished bravery in action on Indian Hill. He knew Allison and Thornbury to be deserving of the rank and expected great things of them in the future, as he did of Carberry drilling his Light Horse on the green about Wallis' house. Technically still only a lieutenant, everyone on the expedition now referred to him as Captain Carberry, and Hartley expected formal commissions for all three to arrive in the next batch of dispatches. Everyone in these ranks recognized them with their new rank despite of what a lackadaisical headquarters called them. And that is all that seemed to matter to the three men anyway. So here on this frontier post their titles were Captain Carberry, Ensign Thornbury, and Ensign Allison. And rightfully so.

"Do you think they are about?" Captain Bush asked, walking up the ladder to Hartley. He stopped at the top of the ladder, gazing over the pointed logs to the woods beyond them.

"Oh, they are there," Hartley said, "skulking and lurking about, watching every move we make." He turned away from the captain, scratching the back of his neck. The fingers of his other hand played nervously about the butt of the pistol stuck in his belt. "I durst wager, fine sir, that there are more

Indians within one hundred and fifty miles of this place and Wyoming, then within like distance from Fort Pitt where so many men are posted. I have written Congress requesting another regiment be sent to Wyoming, lest they all find their frontier borders far closer than what they imagine." Bush rolled an eye towards him.

"I assure you what I have written can be relied upon," Hartley said watching two sergeants stroll through the gate. "What are they about?"

"Just on a stroll to check the brush over there," Bush said, blowing into his hands to warm them against the chill. "I ordered it," he added. "As soon as the barracks are completed I shall have it removed. Swampy ground over there. Walker says it was cleared before the expedition, but it grows fast."

"As does everything in this bush country," Hartley said. A yelp and a shout turned his head quickly back to the sergeants. Stunned, he stared at a painted man smoothly cutting around the crown of one of the men's heads. The other sergeant seemed to have vanished into thin air. "There!" he shouted, raising his pistol and firing a wild shot at the demon. Before the smoke from the pistol cleared the painted devil vanished.

Bush swirled about and flew down the ladder, landing with a thud. He shouted and waved at the men spilling through the gate, directing them to the fallen sergeant.

Dozens of men fanned out immediately into the brush, leaving the frustrated captain standing and running his hands nervously through his hair while he watched the brush. "What the devil!" he called back up to Hartley. "They were just here! Where in the hell could they have gone? And what of the other sergeant?"

"We've a wily foe, Captain," Hartley called back to him, carefully reloading his pistol. "Here in the blink of an eye and gone by the next heartbeat."

The rumble of hooves trampled the ground. Carberry galloped headlong at the head of his Light Horse, saber drawn and with grim determination in his eyes. The horsemen flew by the foot soldiers and burst into the brush and woods beyond it, screaming and hooting as loudly as any

Indian. They soon returned along with the bedazzled foot soldiers, sharing the same baffled look on all their faces.

"They are still about, indeed," Hartley said under his breath. "I fear it shall take more than our feeble numbers to curb their acts against us. I fear for the innocents caught in the midst of this terrible upheaval. Nothing will lessen it but complete destruction of one or the other. This I know. This I fear. God help us all."

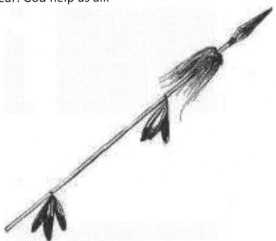

Chapter Sixty-Four

"Well there you be, young Jenkins," Abel Yarington said, grinning at the lieutenant before waving over to the men on the opposite shore of the Susquehanna. "They've secured the tow line." Abel stepped onto his new ferry, looking down at its creaking bottom with concern before nodding at the anxious men standing around the carts aboard it. "Never you mind the creaks, she's new," he said. "She'll be fine after she's broke in like a new coon-dog or woman is all!" Turning, he motioned to a man minding an oxen attached to the other end of the rope after it wound around a huge tree trunk. "Pull!" he ordered the man.

With the sharp crack of a whip the oxen moaned and trudged

ahead, dragging the rope taunt. It sprang from the blue-green water. Abel reached out and grabbed it, making sure it guided easily through eyes of the rail on the side of the ferry. After watching it guide freely through the rail to his satisfaction, he glanced over to the lieutenant standing by a group of canoes filled with well-armed men. "We're ready," he said, "now just get your lot over there ahead of me." He watched the men on the opposite shore eagerly climb back into their canoe and paddle back towards the safe side of the river. "If there be any savage in wait, I'll be pulling hard for this shore again," he added. "You all best make sure it's good and clear. Wave back to me when it's so."

"Sir," Jenkins said, pointing the barrel of his rifle up to the early morning sun, "it is true the day is young, but many a brave soul waits over there to be properly buried, by his own people and not by the cruel hand of nature." He stepped into the canoe waiting for him, nodding to the ferryman. "Best we all set out at the same time, that way we'll all be getting there at the same time and get about our work. I want no time wasted by the timid in case there be trouble. This may be the only day allowed us. I want to get as many buried proper as possible."

Yarington sneered at the insinuation and pulled hard on the tow rope, motioning for the others in the ferry to lend a hand on it. "Then be about your business, sir, and don't be looking over your shoulder for us, for we'll be right behind you, smug rascal. We'll see they're all buried proper." "What's that you say?" Jenkins asked.

"Just do yer part and I'll be sure to do mine," Abel Yarington said. "If you lose your hair, so shall I, but don't be imparting any reluctance on my part, fine sir!"

"Then pull that rope and mind your tongue, you're still in the employ of the army, you know," Jenkins said, waving his arm towards the far shore. With that canoe and ferry swept across the river in one long continuous line. It only slowed once, to meet the men in the canoe paddling from the opposite shore; and then only long enough to tie their canoe to the ferry and pull them aboard it.

In spite of the eagerness of the ferrymen, the ferry slowed just before the shore, letting the canoes land before it. The men in the canoes ignored the ferry. Their eyes remained locked on the trees and bushes lining the shoreline. The hoots, war whoops, and glowing fires from the west shore every night heightened their anxious feelings; plus, the plight of the three Germans killed just a fortnight before their present expedition. The wails and pleas of the poor scalped survivor haunted their minds, sending a loathsome, but familiar chill down their spines. Nonetheless, they fanned out all along the shore and marched forward in perfect military fashion, led by their stern commander. Under the watchful eye of the ferrymen and civilians on the ferry they soon disappeared into the trees and brush.

All aboard the ferry stayed perfectly silent, listening intently for any telltale sounds of distress. After a while rifles rose in some of their hands while others turned around on the rope, ready to pull on it with all their strength in anticipation of a hasty retreat. "You just hold fast," Yarington told them, slapping at their white knuckles clenching the rope. "I meant what I said. If that brash young rowdy loses his hair, so shall I, but I'll not be pulling this ferry away from this shore without taking as many of them across safe as you. If you can't wait then swim, damn you!"

Jenkins suddenly appeared on the shore, waving the ferry to land.

"See," Yarington said, "told you all it'd be fine, and you still got yer hair, ain't ya!"

None of the men laughed at his remark but just pulled steadily on the rope. The forest and trees that had once been so familiar to them now seemed completely foreign, as if conquest had totally changed the very nature of the ground itself. Somehow the horror of what happened at the battle remained embedded in the soul of the earth itself, sending out a lingering warning to all daring to step upon it again. Every man felt the feeling. Every man let it swell in his chest and swallowed hard against it, anxious to be about their duty. They remembered their friends, fathers, and sons, all lying on that field for so long, and the shame of it swept away and subdued their anxious feelings. Their long overdue debt to their brethren overrode fear itself.

Soon the carts creaked forward, surrounded by Jenkins' vigilant soldiers.

Along the way they all stopped to face the ruins of the strong fort they had constructed in a time that seemed so long ago, Forty Fort. Nothing but the hint of one of the cabins within its wall greeted them. Jumbles of logs lay piled in heaps, some half-burned. Others lay split and hacked so as to never rise in defense of Wyoming again. The demolished fort harkened of the complete devastation that lay ahead of them. No one spoke. A whisper would have seemed a yell. The creak of a cart finally broke the stares at the fort and they continued on in a veil of silence.

Alert eyes watched the trees all along the road leading north from the fort. Flankers investigated every suspicious bush along the roadside. Fingers itched to pull the locks of the rifles back in the blinking of an eye. Onward the silent burial party marched, listening, watching, and bracing themselves for the shock of the sight of the carnage that lay ahead of them. Upon reaching the first bend in the road the soldiers in the lead stopped. They raised their hands, signaling for their officer to step forward.

John Jenkins lifted his head high and jutted his chin, silently hoping the remains to be too unrecognizable to identify. He thought it best, gazing up to the sun high in the sky. August had been dry. Perhaps before the September rains the bodies had dried. Perhaps this body would not be that of his friend John Murphy, who he had cheered when they marched out of Forty Fort's gate on that hot July day to collide with a fate too horrible to imagine still, after all this time. He looked to the eyes watching him march to the front, knowing they harbored the same fears. Some of their fathers lay here. Some of their dear friends lay here. Some of their sons lay here.

Arriving to the front of the column, Jenkins looked down at three bodies spaced but a few feet apart, one with an upraised arm in the direction of the fort but a few rods up the road. Had it been this poor soul's last act to reach and pray for someone to deliver them to the fort? But alas, no one came, and here he died, hoping against all odds.

Lowering his rifle, he bent down to the body. Dry, sickly gray, and splotchy yellow skin covered the face staring up to him with empty eye sockets. The clothing draping the dried skin of the skeletons lay mostly in tatters. The sleeve of the upraised arm blew in the breeze. Upon closer look a bit of metal glistened in the sun from one of the fingers of the bony upraised hand. He gently held the hand, slipping a ring from dry cracking skin of the finger. The rigid arm fell loosely to the ground, seeming to give up the ghost for the promise of burial for a body now long overdue to return the dust from whence it came.

He raised the ring to his eyes and twirled it about, carefully looking for any telltale marking on it. Many eyes now watched him.

A gasp rose from one of those standing near him. "That's Perrin Ross's ring!" a man said. Taking a step forward, he knelt next to the lieutenant.

Jenkins handed the ring to the wide-eyed man.

"Sure enough is," the man said, stumbling to his feet and looking to the other two bodies lying close by. He took a few steps next to the body lying face down on the ground. Wisps of sandy brown hair blew in the slight breeze. "And this here's got to be Jeremiah, his brother!" he said, touching the hair. Kneeling down, he carefully rolled the body on its side. The ground somehow preserved enough of the face to make it barely recognizable. The man stared at the face and slowly nodded his head before easing it back down to the ground. He looked over to the other body, and at the great spear still stuck in its ribcage. He shook his head. This body had laid face up too long. Nothing remained of its clothing but ripped shreds of faded linen. Besides, some beast had devoured half of its face. "Don't know who that could have been," the man said. "My God it's worse revisiting this place than it was on that day. These poor souls didn't deserve this."

"No," Jenkins said. "No one did. But we've a lot of ground to cover this day. The battlefield proper is nearly a mile or so up river. We best get these men on a cart and keep going."

Heads nodded and a cart rolled to the bodies.

Bending down two men tried to lift the shriveled body of Lieutenant Ross but fell back in disgust. Arms fell out of dried and loose sockets and the paper-like skin crackled. They stood, took a few steps back, and stared down in horror of what they had done.

"Don't fret," a voice called from behind the party. Abel Yarington strode through the distraught men carrying several two-tined pitchforks in his arms. "Figured they'd be all dried out," he said, looking down at the bodies. "That's why I figured to bring these along." He passed two of the pitchforks to the men. They gently placed one under the upper torso and one under the lower torso, picking up the body in unison. It stayed intact, much to the men's relief.

"Thought you were going to stay back at the ferry?" Jenkins asked Yarington.

"Got bored," he said. "Leastways my man's watching it. It'll be there, don't you fret. But these here's my people too, you know. Wouldn't be right but to lend a helping hand, and anyhow, it seems you all need it. Man should go to the grave in one piece, if'n it can be helped."

"I agree," Jenkins said, "and I'm grateful, too, thank you." "Told ya not to fret," Yarington said. "Now let's get at it! Like ya said, a lot of ground is yet to be covered."

Jenkins walked to the spear sticking in the other man's ribcage and stared at the lone feather dancing in the wind on its handle. Clenching the feather in his hand he angrily ripped it from the spear. Throwing it to the ground he stomped it into the earth before yanking the spear from the man's chest. Gripping it tightly on both ends he brought it down hard on his knee. Its crack sounded loudly across the silent field of carnage. He threw the broken spear to the side and grabbed his rifle, gesturing forward with its barrel. "Keep a sharp eye!" he said. "All of you! If you see anything suspicious shoot and ask questions later. There's no one on this side of the river that we can call friend. This I assure you, so let's get at it!"

The men marched onward, though slowed by the increasing amounts of dried and shriveled bodies. One by one they painstakingly lifted the brittle bodies up by the pitch-forks and loaded them onto the carts. Soon groups of two men with forks strayed all over the fields by the road, accompanied by an equal amount of Jenkins' men to guard them against the ever present enemy. All feared and knew the enemy's prying eyes to be upon them from distant bushes and trees, but nonetheless kept focused on their task, determined to bury as many of the men as they could find.

The groups of scattered men followed the bodies until they funneled around a bridge, bringing the party back together. For a moment they stopped to catch their breath while Jenkins sent a party of men across the bridge to scout the area beyond.

"Carts are getting full already," a civilian with a pitch-fork reported to Jenkins.

Jenkins looked anxiously ahead to his men across the bridge. The dots of cloth in the fields beyond the bridge betokened more bodies lay ahead. He nodded his head at the man and quickly examined one of the carts nearest the bridge. Gazing at the growing heaps of shriveled humanity in the carts he shuddered. He had known each and every one of these souls, and now upon witnessing their remains he felt a sad relief he could not recognize any of their corpses. He bent down, touching the picks and shovels stuck up under one of the carts. "We will have to stop and bury them soon, even before we reach the battlefield proper," he said, standing straight again on the approach of one of his scouts.

"All clear ahead, sir," the man reported.

"Very well," Jenkins said. "Let's get at it again."

Up the road they went, collecting and loading bodies until they lay in great heaps threatening to spill over the top rails of the carts. Noticing the full carts, Jenkins ordered a halt, climbing up a slight knoll by the side of the road. "Here," he said, thumping the butt of his rifle down on the ground, "is where we shall bury them." He looked all around the green grass surrounding the spot and at the tall trees offering some shade. The river stretched below them across a green plain on the right. In all it seemed a proper place for one to spend eternity. Nestled in the valley they so loved in life, it offered a serine place of rest in the comfort of mother earth.

Jenkins himself strutted to a cart, pulling the first pickaxe from underneath it. Without turning to order any of the surrounding men to dig, he strode to the spot, paced a few steps to center himself, and with a great swing struck the pickaxe into the ground. Soon every shovel and pickaxe from the carts joined him in excavating a great wide hole in the earth.

A distinct call, a loud gobble, perked all heads in the direction of the noise. Pickaxes stopped in mid-swing. The gritty sound of shovels moving dirt ceased. Once again the call sounded in the still air. Rifle and musket locks clicked to full cock, rising to the shoulders of Jenkins' alert soldiers.

Jenkins himself stood silent and still. He slowly lowered his pickaxe, intently listening.

The call sounded again, this time further down the road.

More rifles turned towards the noise.

"They ain't no turkeys!" a voice finally announced. "But I bet they're wearing feathers just the same!"

Jenkins struck the pickaxe in the ground with one swift thud and stepped from the hole, reaching for his own long rifle. He lifted the weapon to his shoulder, glaring in the direction of the disturbing sounds.

"Do you want us to check it out?" one of his soldiers asked.

"No," Jenkins said, turning and walking up the road. "If they're there in them woods let them stay there. We're here to collect the dead. I am not going to let the threat of a few of those devils spoil everything! I had a hell of a time convincing Colonel Butler it was safe to come over here as it was, so let's get at it!" He waved a few of his soldiers ahead. "Sergeant Baldwin," he called behind him. "You stay here with about a half dozen or so to guard the diggers while I take the rest ahead."

"Yes sir," Baldwin said, posting his troops in a wide circle around the nervous civilians digging the hole. "You heard the Lieutenant!" he said to the diggers. "Get at it! We ain't going to let them stop us, besides, if'n they was here in any numbers they would have been all over us already. You all know how they is. Daylight's burning! Let's go!"

Some of the diggers grumbled at the brash sergeant but after his glaring eyes caught theirs' they thought better of it. They dug.

Jenkins spread his remaining men out in a wide arc surrounding the carts and burial party plodding up the road. They worked swiftly and steadily, with each man watching out of the corner of his eye while he worked.

Many of them checked the pistols stuck in their belts and twisted them, wanting them loose and ready to fire at a moment's notice. Because of the vastness of the field the party soon split into two; one covering one half of the field while the other covered the other half of it.

Their steps only slowed by the remains of Fort Wintermoot upon sight of a ghastly figure perched among its charred timbers. The burned figure of a man stood slightly bent forward, his hands still clenched in tight fists at his antagonists after all this time. The steel prongs of two-tined pitchforks stuck in his feet, another dangled from the upright corpse from its side. The man no doubt died in defiance of his enemy. The horror of the brave man's death flashed in each of the men's eyes staring at his body in shock and disbelief.

"That's got to be Captain Bidlack," a soldier said. "The story of his torture is true, every damn bit of it, and it looks like more! He fought them so they had to pin him in the flames with pitchforks!" The man's bulging eyes gazed down at the decapitated corpse laying just before the burned ruins of the fort. "And that there's got to be Captain Ransom's body, as well!" He carefully lifted a knee buckle from the decaying corpse's leg. "Them are his fancy knee buckles fer sure, they are," he said. "He was known fer his buckles, now they tell us of his demise, poor, brave soul."

Jenkins stared in blank horror at the bodies. "Collect them," he finally said, remembering the two brave men he had known dearly in life. Apparently they had died as they had lived. His eyes caught the glimpse of the sun lowering just behind the trees to his right. "The day grows long," he said. "We, gentlemen, do not want to be caught on this side of the river at nightfall. Let's get these brave souls buried so they can finally rest in peace."

A cart hurried ahead and two men gently lifted Captain Bidlack's charred body from the ruins. One pulled a prong from the side of his body. "Looks like they stuck him time and time again," he said, "left this one in his hip."

"Yes," Jenkins said, "just get him out of there so we can be on our way." A disgusted grunt turned his head towards a few frustrated men tending to Ransom's body.

"Can't find his head," one of them said to the stern-eyed lieutenant. "Lord knows what they did with it, the bloody rascals! My God, what horrors!"

"Just collect what you can," Jenkins said. "No one can blame you under the circumstances, least of all me. Now let's get these carts full of the dead back to the grave so we have time to cover them properly!"

A call from further back along the road caught their attention. They rushed down a few rods to find men standing around a large rock. They stared in shock at the bodies arranged in a circle around it.

"What is this?" Jenkins asked.

"Torture circle of that half-breed witch Ester," one of them said. He lifted his pitchfork, pointing it towards the rock. Bits of red still shone in the crevices and cracks on its face. On one particular spot bits of dried flesh and other matter lay among a huge splotch of red.

Jenkins slowly paced around the rock, looking down sorrowfully upon the bodies. Though shriveled, several of the skulls appeared to be crushed. Cuts and other signs of misuse showed on their withered and dry skin. What happened here made his stomach lurch. He turned his head away and looked to the river for the longest moment before turning back to the men. "Load them in the carts," he said, overcome with grief. "We must be quick; the sun shall set soon."

One of the party motioned him over to the cart. He looked down at a body to which the man pointed.

"It's Captain Durkee," the man said.

Jenkins looked down at the body, his lower lip raising in disgust. The body's head jutted back, locked in a painful position bearing witness to his dear friend's pain right up to his last moment. The empty, hollow, sockets of his eyes stared towards the heavens. What horror these men witnessed played at the very depths of his soul. He turned his head away, looking with empty eyes to the sky.

"Look to his hand," the man said, thinking his stare needed an explanation. "Captain Durkee lost a finger in life, now it identifies him in death. Poor brave soul."

"They were all brave," Jenkins said through the growing lump in his throat. "Every man on this field was brave and should never be forgotten."

"I'll give you that, Lieutenant," the man said, turning to help lift some of the bodies onto the cart. "I'll grant them all that, fer sure."

The other carts soon converged around the ring. Each man glanced at it with the same disgust before Jenkins ordered the whole party back to the grave site.

Sergeant Baldwin's and his men's eyes lit up at the sight of the returning carts, bearing witness to their growing apprehension since they departed. "The calls are becoming more frequent," the sergeant explained to his lieutenant. "Was getting a bit antsy," he added, looking at his fellows. "All of us was fer sure getting antsy. We're glad to see you."

Jenkins nodded his head, waving the carts past him to the grave. The men, sensing a growing sense of uneasiness on the part of the sentries, worked all the faster at emptying the carts. Soon they placed the last body, Captain Durkee's, unceremoniously atop the others. Shovels promptly went to work covering the huge grave while the anxious eyes of the soldiers watched the woods all around them.

With the last shovel full of dirt, the sound of feet and the backs of shovels tamping down the earth atop the grave turned the guarding soldiers' eyes behind them. The sinking sun grazed the tops of the trees to the west. The shadows of the forest grew deep, seeming to close in on them.

Jenkins strode to the head of the massive grave, sensing the need for someone to say a few words, but feeling anxious for the safety of his command at the same time. "Well," he said, bowing his head and removing his hat, "here they are, many a brave soul whom died for liberty. We knew them all as son, father, grandfather, uncle, brother, and friend. Many of us here marched with them to this very field where they shall forever rest. Let their rest be peaceful, and most of all let their place in our hearts, and our history, never be forgotten. It's true we haven't the time, or perhaps the proper speaker for such an occasion, a preacher or such, but we have done our task here under the threat of the enemy breathing down our necks and howling from the woods. Yes, we all have done our part this day, so let it be to those whom shall reap the rewards of the great and noble sacrifices made here, to commemorate these brave fallen souls, who died for us, and them, with them, their posterity, very much on their minds. For what are all of us but the children in this blinking of time we occupy upon this earth. For all we are in the end, is our children and their children, and so it goes, from time immortal. What happen here should never be forgotten, and I pray most heartedly to God himself that it shall never be. Dear God bless this ground and the bodies lying within it. Kith and kin I pray our posterity shall remember them, and their sacrifices. In that they shall live again. In that the ideals for which they died shall live again. Let all of us never forget, never forget. For that would be a tragedy far greater than any suffering felt by these brave men upon this field. Let their memory live in the hearts of men and the liberty for which they fought shall never be forgotten. I pray this for all standing here and lying in the hollowed earth of this field. No holier spot of ground exists than where defeated valor lies, crowned by mourning's glory. Amen."

With that, the burial party solemnly started marching back to the ferry. Each man walked silently, watching out of the corner of his eye for the same enemy, lest he too be left on this field dead. With feelings of relief tinged with the sorrowful memories of those who had fallen they stepped onto the ferry and filled the canoes.

The beautiful Susquehanna wound before them in the twilight, its swirling waters catching many of the crestfallen eyes watching it wind past them to the far away sea. More eyes turned from the thought of the grave behind them to the hopeful and relieved faces beaming at them from the opposite shore.

Women, children, and their fellow soldiers, all stood waiting anxiously for their safe return. The sight of the new and stout fort rising high on the bank behind the welcoming faces spread smiles of relief across many faces. Perhaps their comrades had not died in vain, they mused. Perhaps they would be remembered after all, and with that their own struggles, also. Perhaps.

But still the memory of that field would never be forgotten as long as they breathed, they promised one another, and they also promised to carry on in the light of the courage shining from their fellows' great sacrifices. No, their memory lived, as Jenkins said, as long as liberty still lived in the hearts of men, great and small. They knew this without a doubt as they spilled from the canoes and ferry to the welcoming arms of their brethren and loved ones. Wyoming lived as long as they breathed. It lived as long as their descendants breathed.

But shadows still cast themselves across the light of liberty, and none the greater in Wyoming than the shadow of the great Six Nations. That shadow penetrated so deep it cast itself across the hope shinning within the souls and the Wyoming settlers, no matter how intense the light of liberty glowed from their hearts.

Could hope alone prevail against the Six Nation's tomahawks?

Could this dreaded *curse of the tomahawk* ever be broken?

Cursed or not by tomahawks clenched in the hands of the great Iroquois Confederacy, the Wyoming people pledged to themselves, their fellow countrymen, and to their posterity, to continue their struggle, urged on by their eternal vision and burgeoning spirit, despite the shadows of gloom. Their spirit, their *American spirit*, fueled by an unquenchable faith in the future and hope of the present, would see them through any difficulties and strife. It had to, for in the end, it is all they had.

"Camp Wioming, Octo. The 3d., 1778

"Colo Hartley takes the opportunity of Returning his thanks to the officers and Soldiers Volluntiers and Others under his command on the Late expedition for their Good Conduct and perfservation during that Tolesome and dangerous March amidst Hunger Wading of River at Midnight.

"Marches no Complaints were heard all was Submifsion and Resignation in Action several Of the Continental officers difhtinguished themselves Capt Boone And Capt Champlane of the Volunters deferve particularly to be Named-Capt Franklin with his Volunters from Wyoming Were Very useful in this Expedition In short with

Very few Exceptions the Whole detachment have acquited themselves With the Highest Reputationand they have this Further Satisfaction to know They have saved the lives of many and served their country Sergt Allison and Sergt thornbury for Action are appointed Enfigns in Colo Hartley's Regiment."

"Oct. 30.

"Dear Genl. (A. Wayne)-You will hear of a splendid expedition we have had up the waters of the Susquehanna-In the actions we had with savages I never saw better choices of ground than they made to attack on- but the last time we outmanouvered them."

"Fate ordained that I was to go to make war on the savages of America instead of on Britain."

"It is hellish work to be fighting those devils." "Your

most obedient and humble servant,

Colo. Thomas Hartley"

"Fort Augusta 7th October 1778

"Sir

"The 5th Inst. Coll. Hartley Returned from an expedition he carryed on against some of the small Indians towns on the North Branch of the Susquehanna, where he was informed there was a party of Indians and Tories Assembled, but they being appraised of Coll. Hartley's march by a party of warriors he met comeing to the West Branch; Whome our People fired uppon and shot their Captain dead uppon which the Indians fled Imeadiatly and alarmed the Towns Coll. Hartley was Bound for, so that they had time to put their families and chief part of their Effects out of the way before he arived there, and when he came to Tiaoga where he took some Tories Prisoners, they informed him of a Town calld Shamung about ten or twelve miles from there where there was a Body of Indians Tories & Regulars in Garrison as good as Six or seven Hundred, Coll. Hartley after Consulting his Officers thought it most Expedient to Return Back without Attempting Shamung, and so after destroying Tiaoga & Shesiken and bringing off fifty or Sixty head of Horned Cattle and some Horses they got there beside several other articles our People Brought them in Canoes.

"In the meantime the Indians was Collecting a party to intercept Coll. Hartley on his march to Wyoming, which they accomplished and fired on our People in front in this side of Wyaloosing, where the Indians had waylay'd our People among a parsel of Rocks as they were marching through a piece of Narrows along the River side, but Coll. Hartleys People Returning the fire briskly made the Enimy Give Way, and marched but a little ways furder when they were fired on again in the Rear and after a brisk fireing on Boath Sides for Some time the Enimy Retreated.

"It must be acknowledged our People beheaved with Courage and Conduct, in bringing off their Wounded all their Cattle and pack Horses, suppose the Enemy followed all the Way to Wyoming and scalped four of Coll. James Murrays men after they arived there, as for a more minute account of this Expedition I Refer you to Coll. Hartleys own letters to the Board of Warr & Executive Council.

"But in the whole it was well Conducted considering the number of men that went with Coll. Hartley, not above two Hundred and fifty which shows that Officers and men beheaved with spirit in bringing with them five Indian scalps besides several more of the Enimy Killed. Col. Hartley's loss was seven killed and Eight wounded includeing those that was killed at Wyoming.

Made in the USA
Middletown, DE
21 September 2023

38906403R00220